Cancer Salves

Cancer Salves

A Botanical Approach to Treatment

INGRID NAIMAN

Seventh Ray Press
SUQUAMISH, WASHINGTON

Copyright 1999 by Ingrid Naiman
Printed in Korea by Pacom Korea 1999, 2004,
2008, 2012, and 2017

Published by

Seventh Ray Press
4708 Tree Ridge Lane, NE
Poulsbo, Washington 98370
E-mail: customer_service@seventhraypress.com
Web site: http://www.cancersalves.com
        http://www.seventhraypress.com

Cataloguing-in-Publication Data
Naiman, Ingrid
    Cancer salves : a botanical approach to treatment /
    Ingrid Naiman.
        p. cm.
    Includes bibliographical references.
    ISBN 1–882834–15–1 (paperback)
    ISBN 1–882834–16–X (hardcover)
    1. Cancer—Alternative treatment. 2. Herbs—
Therapeutic use. 3. Ointments. I. Title.
RC271.H47N35 1999
616.99'4061—dc21   97-46581
                                    CIP

Drawings by Jacqueline Hughes
Illustrations by Colleen McBride
Book Design by David Skolkin
Layout by Ingrid Naiman

Published with the assistance of donations to the
Bodhisattva Trust

*In grateful acknowledgement of the
commitment of those dedicated individuals
who have kept alive a remarkable tradition of
botanical medicine and to the patients who seek
alternatives to conventional cancer treatment.*

Acknowledgments

It is my pleasure to thank Ken Michaelis for first discussing with me his understanding of escharotic treatments of cancer. I would also like to thank Roy Upton of the American Herbalists Guild, Mike A. Flanery of the Lloyd Library and Museum, and Brett Powers of the M. D. Anderson Library for photocopying out-of-print material relevant to escharotics. I am glad to have this opportunity to express my gratitude to Kenny Ausubel, John H. Berge, Jim Callaway, Andrea Conway, Mark Currie, Lucinda Dykes, M.D., Peter Holmes, Rena-Marie Johnson, M.D., Charlie W. Jordan, Ralph W. Moss, Ph.D., Dan Ostrander, Dan Raber, David Sale, Clarissa Smith, Linda van Rigteren, Stephen Snow, M.D., Chad Van Seters, and Karen S. Vaughn for their professional advice and information.

My deep appreciation goes to Colleen McBride for her beautiful drawings of herbs, to Jacqueline Hughes for her medical illustrations, and to Vicki Teague Cooper for her cover design. Thanks also go to Gail Barber, Ellen Kielty, Sue Lerner, Barry Lynes, the late Susan Meares, and Susan Morgan for their painstaking proofreading and editing of the various earlier editions of the book and to Jim Callaway and Sara Klein Ridgley, Ph.D., for going over the version now before you. I would also like to express my respect and gratitude to four people who have aided the birth of this book: Bill Blitz, the original designer of my web site (http://www.cancersalves.com); David Skolkin, designer of this book; Jane Heimlich, trusted advisor and author of the focused foreword to this book; and Michael Tierra, fellow educator whose challenges forced exacting attention to every detail.

Though I have chosen not to reveal the names of the persons who commented on their use of the salves and boluses, I would like to thank them for sharing their experiences and thereby making it possible for me to write this book. Finally, it goes without saying that this book would not have seen the light of day had it not been for the enthusiastic feedback of the many practitioners and patients who have used these treatments in their own quests for cure.

Ingrid Naiman

Contents

Foreword

I FIRST LEARNED ABOUT CANCER SALVES while researching my book, *What Your Doctor Won't Tell You* (HarperCollins, 1990.) A breast cancer patient told me she credited her recovery to these salves. Her doctor, the late H. Ray Evers, M.D., a much loved and respected pioneer in alternative medicine, had applied the black and yellow salves. After one month, she expelled the malignant tumor.

Seven years later, to my surprise, I received a phone call from a Cincinnati Methodist minister, Ernest Bromley, who had been diagnosed with a malignant tumor close to his right ear. Rejecting surgery, which he was told might destroy his hearing and ability to swallow, Bromley learned about the black and yellow salves from my book. He later obtained the salves and used them. After close to a month of treatment, he expelled numerous tumors. A follow-up CT scan detected no malignancy.

Naturally, I was pleased to learn about Bromley's successful experience with the salves, and my part in his story. At the same time, I was decidedly uneasy about these cancer salves and my role in writing about them. As a long-time advocate of alternative medicine, I have prided myself on bringing safe and effective cancer treatments to readers' attention. With Dr. Evers' demise, I knew of no other practitioner using this treatment. To my knowledge, no documentation attesting to the salves' efficacy or safety existed. Were these salves safe for patients to use without professional supervision? Would they produce the effects patients hoped for? My only source of information about the salves was Ken Michaelis, St. Louisville, Ohio, a trusted distributor of herbal products. "I can't tell you how they work," he said. All he knew was that the salves were derived from an herbal formula used by Native Americans.

I was troubled by such uncertainties. Imagine my delight, the summer of '94, to receive an advance copy of *Cancer Salves: A Botanical Approach to Treatment*, by Dr. Ingrid

Naiman, a medical philosopher and cancer counselor. Dipping into the book, *Cancer Salves*, my excitement mounted. This book was so good! I warmed immediately to the author's measured assessment of the salves. The salves are not cures for cancer, she writes. Naiman firmly believes that only by addressing "the underlying and often hidden causes of cancer" can one effect a cure. That said, the author describes cancer salves as "a method for removing tumors that is far less invasive and mutilating" than the standard methods employed today.

If you, like myself, are a seeker of information about alternative medicine, in this book you'll find little known but vital information that the author has gathered with painstaking care. You may be surprised, as I was, to discover that cancer salves have a rich history that includes investigations by such visionaries as Hippocrates and Hildegard of Bingen. I discovered that these salves were not solely used by Native American healers. They were employed by several eminent 19th and early 20th century physicians; one of these physicians was instrumental in the founding of the New York Academy of Medicine.

Naiman provides more than historical lore. In *Cancer Salves*, she renders the great service of collecting formulas for preparing the salves that were utilized by illustrious practitioners through the Ages.

If you've been diagnosed with cancer, or know someone who has, this book will be enormously helpful. Practitioners, too, will find it useful treating in cancer patients. In this comprehensive book, you will learn about different types of cancer salves, methods used by outstanding practitioners, and case histories and testimonials from users. Color photos graphically illustrate the "application process" (a strong stomach required, please!) She also thoroughly addresses the fear of recurrence and metastasis as well as the issue of pain and suggests natural ways to reduce this major obstacle to the treatment.

The all-important question, "Do I need supervision when using the salves," and many other concerns, are covered in the "Answers to Questions" section.

Today, a growing number of practitioners in the U.S. and Europe confer with Naiman about the use of cancer salves. With this book, you have the author's wealth of experience and knowledge, both practical and philosophical, at your finger tips. Above all, you will sense a caring empathetic healer at your side.

JANE HEIMLICH
Author of *What Your Doctor Won't Tell You*
Cincinnati, November 1997

Preface to the Third Edition

THOUGH I AM NOT A MEDICAL DOCTOR and do not therefore treat people for cancer, I do counsel people who are ill, often seriously so. In 1990, I heard about a Native American method of cancer treatment involving the external use of herbal salves or pastes that "pull" tumors out of the body. What follows is the report of the trail I have traced. It is my sincere hope that you find it both fascinating and healing.

INGRID NAIMAN
Santa Fe, Summer 1997

*P*reface to the Second Edition

TRY AS I MIGHT, I have been unable to turn my back on the cancer salves, elixirs, and herbal boluses since first learning about them in 1990. Little by little, more information has come my way. At first I heard vague stories about Native American treatments that, according to an ancient tradition, had been passed along on the deathbed of an elder who had himself or herself been guarding the secret of these botanical treatments. Then, odd passages of old herb books, rare and compelling research papers, anecdotal stories, and variations of the formulae began reaching me. Once interested, more details started coming to my attention—and my own understanding of the treatment developed accordingly. I am not a physician, but I began to feel that I am a repository for obscure fragments of an almost lost approach to cancer treatment that needs serious investigation.

In preparing this edition for publication, I tried to define my own relationship both to cancer and to the approaches to its treatment covered in this book. I am what might be called a "medical philosopher." My interest, since childhood, has been in why people become ill and why certain people develop one form of illness and others another. How to deal with the illnesses once they occur has never been my primary focus; but it does seem to me that when a condition is truly understood and healing strategies are employed that actually impact the causes of disease, there is more probability of cure. As such, the herbal approaches covered in this book fall somewhat short of my personal ideal since, for the most part, they address the appearance rather than the underlying and often hidden causes of cancer. Nevertheless, the salves constitute a way of removing tumors that is far less invasive and mutilating than the methods that are today standard—and, if for no other reason, they warrant investigation.

MY PHILOSOPHY OF HEALING

I have been a psychospiritual and health consultant for years. I know the frustration, the desperation, and the suffering of cancer patients —and of those who love them. I also know that, as the disease progresses and ever more drastic treatments are recommended, a quite understandable sense of futility and/or powerlessness can arise. I see, too, that as a civilization, we are at a crossroads where medicine and healing are concerned; we might even be at a new point in our concepts of life and death. In this philosophical area, I have strong beliefs. Among these is a firm conviction that one's body is one's own. It is, therefore, not only one's own responsibility to care for one's body, but it is also within one's rights to use whatever approaches to its maintenance one wishes. Since in order to care for oneself properly it is necessary to be well-informed, I believe that we have a right to the knowledge that can enhance our grasp of what our needs and our options are.

Knowledge can be a double-edged sword. It is empowering if individuals are able to make informed judgments about what would support their own best interests; it is frustrating when reliable information is lacking, and weakening if sound ideas are ignored. Conventional medicine has little better than stock answers for the serious questions faced by persons with life-threatening illnesses. Often as not, patients are told how their conditions should be treated but not what their prognoses might be with those treatments—nor what the short- and long-term side effects of the treatments are. In most instances, survival, as understood from the scientific side, is a numbers game measured in years rather than cure. In reality, modern medicine probably does not have anything approaching a genuine cure for cancer.

Moreover, the various blood and tissue tests conducted on patients do not solve either their medical or personal dilemmas, such as their deeper life or death issues. Attachments to life as it is known and to the people who are important to them, concerns about responsibilities, and doubts about life after death are not discussed—nor are the alternative treatments that may enhance their quality of life or survival. Patients are left to grapple with these matters on their own. I believe that adequate resolution of these important matters might be more crucial to survival than the actual treatments elected.

For me, life and death are inner issues while treatments are outer decisions—based, hopefully, on the best possible use and interpretation of available information. My experience with many patients seeking alternative treatments is that they are exhausted by their quests for cure, depressed by the impersonality and horror of their experiences, and sometimes ambivalent as to whether or not they can actually undergo additional efforts to recover— especially if such involve more pain and mutilation. Throughout the often long course of illness, patients are called upon to sacrifice their feelings to bizarre technology that frequently fails to cure cancer. Weakened by disease and invasive procedures, further effort and stoicism often seem impossible, even the alternative measures, since lack of physician supervision means that patients must be both self-motivated and self-disciplined if they are to assume primary responsibility for treatment.

INVOLVEMENT

Cancer patients often feel that they are victims. They feel themselves to be victims of the social dynamics operating in their lives, victims of brutal medical procedures, and victims of a fate they neither understand nor appreciate. Cancer is a dreaded disease. Dealing with its discovery and facing the treatments can be frightening; but, in my opinion, neglecting the causes is nearly certain to be fatal and, towards the end anyway, more terrifying than the treatments.

Modern research on the effects of thought and emotion on health, the so-called body-mind connection, is unequivocal: what happens in the body, particularly with the immune system, is inseparable from the more difficult-to-measure subtleties and secrets of the mind and emotions. Once a body-mind connection has been made, a powerful sense of involvement arises in all that is happening, both to the body and within the psyche. With such realizations comes another challenge, one that is often resisted by patients. When a patient already feels himself or herself to be a victim, to suggest that he or she may have participated in the creation of his or her realities, whether social or medical, may feel like insult added to injury. Finding the body-mind connection does not, however, have to be a guilt trip; it can be an adventure.

We have been acculturated to believing in physical causes for what seem to be physical conditions. In the case of cancer, exposure to specific environmental hazards, demographic and genetic risk factors, and perhaps diet are but a few of the presumed causes. In these and similar lines of inquiry, answers to such truly important questions as "Why me?" and "Why now?" are not found. Since the real cure is probably not far from the cause, I have, in my other writings, proposed an entirely different attitude and approach to cancer and its treatment.

It may seem healthy for a victim to resist the notion that feelings or hidden facets of the psychospiritual nature contribute to illness, yet virtually all specialists in such matters insist that our experiences, and how we react to those experiences, play a part in our wellness or lack thereof. Add me to the list of those who believe that no cure is ever complete, even when the symptoms seem to go away, unless the causes of the disease have been eliminated. Many of these causes are deep; but, in my estimation, they magnetize the very experiences we are consciously determined to avoid. I see a need for communication between the inner and outer voices, between the subjective and objective realities. Thus, if fear of pain, of the unknown, or of death are part of the disease experience, the sorrows and mysteries of our being need also to be explored and brought into alignment with the more linear aims that guide our medical decisions.

Cancer patients have often told me that they are afraid of what they might uncover if they looked deeper within themselves. My response is that where life is at stake, pulling a sheet over the head is not a particularly effective response. It is "bite the bullet" time. Biting the bullet may help to restore whatever sense there is that control over life has been eroded. Moreover, it is possible that looking within is inescapable, that it will either occur as a life saving investigation (in this dimension) or as part of the death experience.

In my view, blind obedience to orthodoxy is not a practical response to cancer. In fact, it may be part of the victim syndrome whereas using one's predicament to declare one's right to be true to oneself may be the most efficacious course. Ultimately, life is an experience. Experiences are objective: birth, growth, graduation, career, marriage, birth of children and grandchildren, health, and ultimately death. Experiences are also subjective: happy or sad, exhilarating or frightening, rewarding or challenging, enriching or discouraging. It is my position that the processes, including the crises, that lead us where we are going are as important as the goals themselves. What we experience and what we feel are at least equal in meaning to what we achieve outwardly. I resist the notion that life can be evaluated using the same quantitative measures used in science. Life has intangible experiential components as well as a spiritual essence. Elsewhere I have written extensively on these more philosophical matters, but this book is intended to be practical. Nevertheless, in right conscience, I cannot consider anything practical if it ignores the deeper aspects of existence, those that transcend pathology and medicine.

These beliefs haunted me when someone very dear to me died in 1993. I lost all interest in the salves and resumed my brooding on the meaning of existence. As said, I am a medical philosopher. On one level, I wanted to believe that my friend's death was not necessary; on another, I had to know what really determines whether a person is to continue living for some time to come or to die. I abandoned interest in all physical aspects of life, except my own nutrition, and spent my time in contemplation. I consulted fifteen to twenty psychics, channels, and clairvoyants, listened to their various insights, and wound up writing a book on fate rather than on diet and herbs.

Meanwhile, the telephone did not stop ringing. Responding to the mention of the earlier version of this book in *Options* by Richard Walters, desperate people begged me to guide them to the use of the salve. This was agony for me. Though I did not want to turn my back on anyone who was ill, I was not interested in anything but the answers to life's truly big question: "Why?"

COMPREHENSIVE RESPONSE TO CANCER

As I write this today, I want to say what I think people with cancer need to know: there are many alternative approaches to the treatment of cancer. Since meeting my first cancer patient some twenty-five years ago, I have heard hundreds and hundreds of stories. I have seen people spend years chasing one hope after another, some evidently recovering and others not.

When my friend died, I was accused of having given her false hope. The alternative— what her doctor had given her—was false despair. The fact is that she lived much longer than originally forecast, and she lived a life of remarkable quality until the very end, until the last few weeks.

Perhaps the perfect position would have been totally neutral, neither hope nor despair; but this is not realistic. We know now, without a shadow of a doubt, that the immune system responds to emotions, that hope stimulates the immune system, and that despair inhibits the body's ability to generate its own healing. We also know that chemotherapy is not the miracle humanity had hoped, that surgery is maiming, and that radiation may cause secondary cancers. Patients are entitled to alternatives. The escharotic salves were described by one doctor as a blend of chemotherapy and surgery and by my friend as "the salve from hell." They are radical, not "friendly," but they are often effective.

THE SALVES

In my opinion, the salves, elixirs, and boluses are not cures for cancer, but they are reasonable alternatives to the procedures and protocols offered by modern science. If used properly, *and this is a most important point*, they do not have harmful side effects. Moreover, they can often be used in situations that are regarded as hopeless, for example, cases in which the tumors are inoperable. They are perhaps the ideal options when situations do not seem immediately dangerous, when time is not such an urgent concern, and when some experimental efforts are worth trying before more drastic and irreversible measures are considered.

We are living in a time in which many body parts are regarded as expendable. While those parts may not be vital, they do have func-

tions and they may also be cherished. The thyroid, breasts, womb, and prostate are all intrinsic parts of our expression as humans. Life without such parts often seems less full. Moreover, almost no one wants to be operated on or to lose parts of himself or herself. Some people feel stigmatized by the loss of certain parts of their bodies, and there is often a genuine need for grieving for the losses felt by those who have sacrificed parts of themselves to the surgeon's knife. This is true regardless of whether the organ was part of one's normal physiological functioning or of one's sexual identity.

Personally, I am devoted to the concept of wholeness—wholeness of body, of character, of self expression, and of Spirit. I believe we are life incarnate and that our survival depends on a proper receptivity to inspiration as well as correct interpretation and acceptance of experience. Substances do not explain human existence; we are not merely two-thirds water plus some chemicals. We are complex individuals with unique histories and experiences, and with reactions to those experiences that are held in vast memory vaults deep in our psyches.

There is really nothing in medical science that adequately explains life. Life is not a pulse or a brain wave. It is more mysterious than anatomy and physiology make it out to be. Life is Divine. Life is what unites us with Creation. When we are living, we are participating in Creation; but what is this Creation? Ultimately, it is the expression of Divine Idea, the movement of Spirit in Reality.

I believe that we each have a destiny, one bestowed by our Creator; but, for me, *fate* and *destiny* are not synonymous terms. Destiny is the dynamic manifestation of our spiritual goals. Before we come to the point at which we begin to recognize and fulfill our destinies, we have many experiences. These experiences are essentially emotional, not mental or physical. Certainly we may have feelings about ideas or about incidents that are physical; but experience itself is emotional, and, like the screaming or crying of infants, all experience needs understanding response, validation, and acceptance.

The moment is best understood as the point where destiny and experience intersect, and any given moment may be more spiritual or more emotional, more dynamic or more reflective, more transcendental or more personal.

The Cause of Cancer

I believe that cancer is a disease of congestion in the experiential realm. When emotions are not processed, they tend to stand still, to freeze, and eventually to paralyze the life energies that are trying to express themselves through the personality. Why do emotions freeze? They do so when there is a belief that the movement or expression of the feelings would be catastrophic. If a patient believes his or her truth will be ignored or trivialized, his or her anger met with greater rage, his or her grief glossed over, the patient is likely to suppress movement of his or her feelings until all spontaneity, emotional honesty, and metabolic functioning are impaired. These views do not imply that wild and reckless expression is essential to health, merely that acknowledgment of deeply-held, personal truths is crucial to existence.

Life is dual: it is spiritual and physical. Inspiration from Spirit infuses space with living essence, and the forms that are thus built hold both substance (tissues) and memories of all that has been experienced while living. Without the cooperation of mind and Spirit with body and feelings, no balance is possible, and the viability of the joint creation is jeopardized.

Cancer patients tend to have inordinately developed senses of responsibility; but what is this concept of duty except "mind over matter?" Until there is as much reverence for matter, which includes both form and feelings, as there is for mind, there will be impaired vitality of the body that has to contain all the ideas, objectives, and inspiration duty imposes on it. Life is meant to be enriching, flowing, and eternal—not restricted and impaired by concepts of what is permissible and what is not. What is not allowed to move is suppressed, and I would maintain that this suppression is the real cause of death by cancer.

Thus, while I would indeed support the relief of bodily ills by appropriate physical measures, in the quest for wholeness, I would never neglect my own truths, either the transpersonal or the emotional. Take this advice and read the rest with a measure of caution as to the extent to which reliance can be placed on physical measures alone.

May God the Father and the Divine Mother bless you and protect you and lead you to wholeness, wellness, and holiness.

Ingrid Naiman
Cundiyo, June 8, 1994

*A*uthors Statement

IN RECENT YEARS, the quality of our environment and food has deteriorated, and stress—
which leads to medical and emotional crises
—has crescendoed out of control. During this
same time frame, the incidence of cancer has
increased. Younger and younger patients are
discovering that they are harboring malignancies. Though sophisticated technology may be
facilitating earlier diagnosis, the ability to cure
cancer has not kept pace with either the hazards
affecting survival or the advances experienced
in certain areas of medicine. Many treatments
today prescribed for cancer have both grievous
side effects and questionable success.

There have been two forces impelling me
to present information on the use of salves,
elixirs, and boluses in the treatment of cancer:

• First, those who have cancer have alternatives to conventional treatment. The practices described in the pages that follow have
survived many fashions in medicine. The methods are hundreds, perhaps thousands, of years

old; and as with so many medicines offered by
Nature, these botanical treatments for cancer
are relatively free of side effects.

• Second, when I began to see and experience the action of these traditional remedies, I
felt a need to do my part to preserve a knowledge of their use. The fact that this effort has
also made it possible to assist, in however
modest a way, the fascinating and tireless work
of ethnobotanists and medical anthropologists
is simply a bonus for one such as myself who is
both curious and eclectic.

Salves and boluses are an alternative many
persons with cancer may want to consider.
When used in conjunction with a proper diet,
adjunctive herbal remedies, and sensible life
style adjustments, they offer a promising holistic approach to wide scale suffering, mutilation, and perhaps even to death.

PART ONE

The Salves

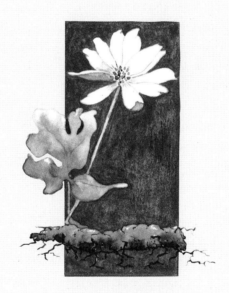

BLOODROOT
Sanguinaria canadensis

Definitions

Some of the terms used in this book will be new for some readers. Each time a technical term is used, an effort to define it has been made by placing a sidebar near the place where the term is first used in the text.

In the title, I have used the term "salves" because many of the people who produce the products described in this book call their products salves. Technically, a salve is an ointment that contains something oily. As such, some of the herbal remedies discussed in this book are actually pastes, not salves. In any event, the majority of the preparations discussed in this book are escharotics, caustic compounds that are applied externally, directly to the skin. Moreover, unlike certain similar products, none of the preparations covered in this book are rubbed into the skin. They are simply applied topically, usually rather thickly. The usages of the words for the purposes of this book are to the right.

Paste: a preparation of herbs and other substances, such as flour, water, ashes, zinc chloride, or minerals. The consistency of the mixture is usually somewhat thick but malleable.

Salve: an ointment using oil or fat. Salves tend to penetrate better than pastes; however, because of their oiliness, they also tend to spread when warmed by the heat of the body.

Plaster: an oil or wax-based medication. It is thick, soft, and easy to handle. The effects of plasters are gradual so these types of applications are used where long-term benefits are sought, especially where the object is pain relief, disinfection, or promotion of tissue growth.

Poultice: similar to a plaster except that the herbs may be in a water or tincture base. Poultices are sometimes called cataplasms. Their action is generally faster than that of a plaster. They can be used to reduce inflammation and infection, to stimulate circulation, to relieve pain or spasms, or to draw off morbid discharges.

Salves

An Historical Overview

A DINOSAUR FOSSIL WITH BONE CANCER—a remnant of a species that roamed the earth for 150 million years before becoming extinct 65 million years ago—was discovered in Wyoming. Cancer of the thigh bone was found in the remains of an anthropoid, estimated to be a million years old, excavated in Java in 1891. Mummified remains of Egyptian pharaohs discovered in the Great Pyramid of Gizeh also showed evidence of bone cancer. Although cancer of other types must also have existed in ages past, the proof would long since have vanished. Bones survive, and from their silent testimony, we can be certain that we who live on this Earth have been suffering from cancer and seeking a cure for it for a long, long time.

Today cancer is probably the most dreaded disease on the Planet. It strikes young and old of all Nations, animals as well as people, and leaves in its wake tragic suffering and emptiness. The presentation that follows traces the history of one particular approach to cancer treatment that seems, despite its antiquity, to remain relevant—especially in light of the failure of modern medicine to affect cancer survival in any meaningful way.

Among the most ancient cures are a variety of escharotic salves and pastes that are applied externally for the treatment of visible and palpable cancers. These treatments, along with surgery, have been the primary methods of treating cancer for at least the last 2,500 years. The Hindu epic Ramayana (circa 500 B.C.) refers to an arsenic paste. Hippocrates, (460–377 B.C.), the Father of Modern Medicine, combined caustics (substances that burn) with cautery (use of heated objects, such as iron instruments, that burn).

Medicine and science are not necessarily progressing in a straight line towards enlightenment. Beliefs and theories have their advocates and cycles. Hippocrates, who gave us the word *carcinoma*, preferred caustics. In the early centuries after Christ, the Roman Celsus (1st century A.D.) and Greek Galen (c. 130–200 A.D.) were inclined towards surgery. Celsus is believed to have been the first in history to

ESCHAROTIC
A caustic substance (acid or base) that causes a chemical reaction with tissue. The reaction is usually attended by heat, itching, and burning and results in the destruction of the reactive tissue.

CAUSTIC
A substance that burns.

CAUTERY
The use of a hot instrument to destroy tissue.

have operated on cancer and ligated blood vessels. A few centuries after Celsus, European medicine became dominated by Islam which forbade surgery. So, from the sixth century through the Middle Ages, herbal medicine in the West achieved great heights. Then, the Inquisition put a virtual end to botanical practices in Europe.

During the Renaissance, methods of cancer treatment again became the subject of debate. The famous Italian anatomist Gabriel Fallopius (1523–1562), renowned for his description of the fallopian tube and his skill as a surgeon, was superintendent of the Padua botanical gardens and much interested in the medicinal properties of plants. Fallopius used caustics. However, towards the end of the Renaissance, surgeons had come to associate caustic treatments of cancer with the increasingly unfashionable *humoral* theories of disease taught by Hippocrates and Galen who though divided on how best to treat cancer— shared the belief that cancer was caused by an increase in black bile, the melancholic humor. Thus, a century after Fallopius, Henri Ledran (1685–1770) rejected the humoral theories— and in so doing tended to negate the psychosomatic basis of disease, the relationship of mood or *humor* to illness. Ledran advocated surgery, this despite the fact that the survival rate remained under five percent for more than another century and despite his recognition of the *lymphatic* system and its possible role in metastases.[1] In other words, even though it had been known since the time of Celsus that cancer can metastasize and thus become a systemic rather than local condition, Ledran put his stock in surgery rather than pastes and ointments and their adjunctive internal tonics.

The escharotic treatments did not, however, disappear. Had they vanished, they would, at this time, only be of interest to archivists. However, the fact that their use persists alongside modern conventional treatments suggests that, at least among certain patients and health care professionals, herbal salve use is regarded as an effective way of dealing with cancer. Even the most vehement opponents of escharotic treatments of cancer have often been forced to acknowledge their efficacy, faulting them mainly for their antiquity rather than failure to perform as required. In short, unlike most traditional botanic remedies, the claims are based not only on vague testimonials but also on empirical evidence and trials repeated over at least the last two hundred and fifty years.

As we are about to discover, many of the herbal cancer treatments were shrouded in secretiveness or conflict. Among those who challenged their use, it would appear that persecution was based more on greed for patents than clinical shortcomings, this whether in eighteenth century London or twentieth century America. Centuries of innuendo and legal conflicts have not, however, managed to suppress the use of the pastes.

What follows is an account of these botanical treatments for cancer and their various proponents from the twelfth century to the present.

HILDEGARD OF BINGEN
12th Century

Hildegard of Bingen, a twelfth century German mystic, was by all accounts an extraordinary healer and visionary. Though proper diet was the foundation of her preventative medicine, she saw faith as an equal source of protection against illness. A proper attitude and absence of spiritual risk factors, such as doubt, were considered by Hildegard to be essential to true health. The monasteries of her day catalogued hundreds of herbal remedies; however, Hildegard's insights were original and came straight from her visions.

> *In all creation, trees, plants, animals, and gem stones, there are hidden secret powers which no person can know of unless they are revealed by God.* [2]

Hildegard is the first historic figure whose cancer salve has been studied in modern times. Her recipe utilized the expressed juice of violets (*Viola spp.*), olive oil, and billy goat tallow. She said that the viruses (*vermes*) that were devouring the patient would die when they tasted the salve. Interestingly, a few years ago, 1989, when the U. S. Food and Drug Administration (FDA) requested that chaparral be withdrawn from the market, some herbalists substituted violets for this familiar Native American cancer remedy.

It is worth noting that although a viral link to human cancers remains the subject of much investigation, Hildegard offered this insight eight hundred years ago. She and her mystic brothers in Tibet apparently shared a kind of clairvoyance that has never been replaced by the microscope. With their divine sight, they saw tiny creatures that have only barely begun to be described by science.

In addition to her violet salve, Hildegard described a complex elixir[a] based on duckweed (*Lemna minor*) that was to be used to protect against cancer. She also prescribed various yarrow beverages to prevent metastases.

ELIXIR
A tonic, usually rejuvenative and sweet.

THE INQUISITION
1231–1834

The history of cancer treatment in Europe cannot be fully understood without reference to the Inquisition. The Holy Office was established in the thirteenth century to root out heretics, people who did not subscribe to the views of the Church. In order to maintain the purity of theological tenets, lay persons were not permitted to study the Bible. By the fifteenth century, control of beliefs extended to all thought, including medicine, which at that time was largely a monastic pursuit, not, as today, a scientific discipline taught in secular universities and sponsored by large corporations. Given the influence of religion on medical thought, it cannot be a surprise that, in the Middle Ages, illness was generally regarded as a manifestation of sin. As such, ashamed and guilt-ridden patients often failed to report their early symptoms. When their conditions

---

[a] The formula for this is given in appendix B, page 187.

finally required medical intervention, doctors tended to withhold pain relievers so that patients could suffer and thereby fully atone for their iniquities. It was a desperate and dark time in the annals of Western medicine.

The extent of the enmeshment of church and state in those sorry times can be understood by relating the tribulations of Jacoba Felicie, an educated woman in a Dark Age. Felicie was brought to trial by the Faculty of Medicine at the University of Paris in 1322. She was accused of curing her patients of internal illnesses and wounds and of visiting the sick. Witnesses testified that after university-trained physicians had failed to cure them, they had been healed by Felicie. The issue was then, as today, not results but conformity to an authoritarian system that decided what is orthodox and what is not.

Under the Auto-Da-Fé (Act of Faith), the first Inquisition execution took place in 1481, in Seville, during the incumbency of the most feared of all Grand Inquisitors, Tomás de Torquemada. The official guidebook for persecution during the Inquisition was the *Malleus Maleficarum* (1486) written by two Dominican monks, Heinrich Kramer and Jakob Sprenger, who in today's world would be advised to undergo therapy for their sadism. Though women and homosexuals were the main targets of the *Malleus Maleficarum*, it was midwives who were most severely attacked.

> *Midwives cause the greatest damage, either killing children or sacrilegiously offering them to devils . . . The greatest injury to the Faith is done by midwives, and this is made clearer than daylight itself by the confessions of some who were afterwards burned.* [3]

The confessions that were used as evidence against the accused were, as we know, extorted from persons who were subjected to the most extreme tortures ever catalogued in Christendom. During the Inquisition's reign of terror, it is estimated that as many as nine million persons, mostly women, were burned at the stake, often for such crimes as practicing herbal medicine—because healing interfered with the punishments disease was inflicting on the suffering. According to the *Malleus Maleficarum*, healing is a crime committed by witches who must be put to death for their deeds. The *Malleus Maleficarum* called for the eradication of the knowledge of herbal healing—mainly on the grounds that reliance on such measures reduces our dependence on God.

The pursuit of knowledge encountered obstacles even after the advent of the Renaissance. Nostradamus (1503-1566) was a practicing physician during the sixteenth century. He was treating the bubonic plague with little pills containing rose petals. He was accused of possession of books banned by the Church. He was hauled before the Inquisition but rescued by royal intervention as he was a great favorite of Catherine de' Medici, queen of France but daughter of the leading patron of the Italian Renaissance Lorenzo de' Medici, whom Pope Sixtus IV had tried to have assassinated. Despite the efforts of secret societies, such as that to which Nostradamus belonged, to preserve ancient knowledge, European herbal traditions were nearly eradicated by the Inquisition.

Though Galileo Galilei (1564–1642) abandoned his medical studies to pursue mathematics and philosophy, his story provides us with an excellent example of thought control and persecution in the seventeenth century. Galileo was brought before the Inquisition for supporting the revolutionary Copernican view of astronomy; and, in 1616, he was ordered not to discuss Copernicanism. When the cardinal who first brought charges against him died, Galileo published his heretical views and, in 1633, was sentenced to life imprisonment. Though his sentence was commuted to house arrest, the trial documents were not published until 1870. Acknowledgment of error by a Papal commission was only accorded in October 1992!

In today's world, the Inquisition's methods and objectives are difficult to understand. The tortures and executions in Europe prevailed for more than three hundred years, the same time period that Europeans were colonizing the Americas and other parts of the world that explorers had discovered. During this errant time, it was not unusual for the entire female population of a town, including children and the elderly, to be exterminated by the Church. The Inquisition was not fully suppressed until 1834.

Between war, plague, and the Church, life in Europe was, for many centuries, precarious. With genocide and death everywhere, conditions must have been nothing short of horrific.

What is astonishing is that the Renaissance neither liberated nor enlightened to the extent often imagined. It did, perhaps, inaugurate an age of inquiry, but older ways were supplanted by a new science that remained as unfriendly to tradition as it was to the environment. In such an uncongenial intellectual atmosphere, natural medicine had few exponents. It is therefore to the Americas and its Native American medicine men and women that we look to explain the revival of interest in botanic medicine, including escharotic cancer treatments.

The New World
Seventeenth Century

The earliest settlers who landed on the Atlantic shores had some knowledge of European remedies, but as they pushed westward they necessarily had to resort to the indigenous medicines, the properties of which could most readily be learned from the Indians.

VIRGIL J. VOGEL,
American Indian Medicine, p. 125.

The discovery of the New World launched a booming two-way trade between the Colonies and Europe. Exchange flourished not only in slaves, sugar, and tobacco, but also in herbs. Review of historically preserved European herbal recipes reveals that ingredients were imported from such faraway places as India and Sri Lanka as well as the New World.

When Europeans began colonizing the New World, they encountered illnesses that were not familiar to them and flora whose uses they did not know. Especially among the French, who saw the Indians as trading partners rather than as savages to be subjugated, there was considerable fraternization with Native American medicine men. In the seventeenth century alone, scores of papers were published on nonsurgical tumor removal using poultices, plasters, and ointments containing New World herbs.

> Many of the early botanic physicians professed to have absorbed their knowledge directly from contact with the Indians. Some of them had indeed, by reason of captivity, trade, or other occasion for proximity with the natives, found opportunities to learn the red man's procedure and remedies. Some claimed to be at least partly of Indian descent. It was through these men that some of the Indian medical remedies passed to the whites.[4]

Vogel goes on to quote C. A. Browne as saying that, although many remedies were "slow in obtaining official recognition . . . the popularity of some of the Indian remedies, when once physicians began to describe them, became so great in some cases as almost to cause extinction of the plant."

Where cancer salves were concerned, bloodroot was by far the most popular ingredient. However, cancer poultices used a wide variety of ingredients ranging from roasted red onions to red clover. Heritage from Native Americans is evident even today: when I took some film for use in this book to a photo laboratory, the clerk asked if the picture had been taken of someone who had employed the same onion treatment for cancer that her family had been using for generations. I was eventually to find that this remedy is extremely popular among lay practitioners.

Aversion to the knife, fear of surgery and mutilation, and a sincere desire for less drastic ways to treat cancer have caused many people throughout history to develop exceptional skill in the use of relatively safer botanic medicines.

RICHARD GUY, SURGEON
1759

Richard Guy, doctor and member of a prestigious corporation of surgeons in London, was famous for his treatment of "scirrhous tumors and cancer." When he heard of a lay treatment using poultices, he was, as might be expected, skeptical about the claims made for the treatment. His doubts, however, turned to wonder when he saw reversals of the fates of patients within weeks after applying the poultice. For a substantial sum, Guy purchased the formula from a family named Plunkett who had been guarding the secret treatment for a century.[5] In 1759 he published a paper describing one hundred cures using this new nonsurgical method.

Guy reported his findings meticulously, along with criticisms of methods he found ineffective. His powers of observation were remarkable by any standard, ancient or modern, and his writing was eloquent.

> Whosoever reflects, that the breasts are composed of almost innumerable small glands, lymphatic and lactiferous ducts, blood vessels, nerves, membranes, etc. all of the most delicate texture and most exquisite sensibility, will not wonder at their being more particularly susceptible of morbid afflictions, as well from internal as external causes.[6]

The terminology used by pre-modern specialists in botanic medicine to describe cancer processes and their treatment evidences awareness that tumors have roots that need to be removed if recurrences are to be avoided. Thus, many of their processes involved the separation of the tumors from their supporting tissues. When the tumors were thus removed, they were often seen to have spider-like protrusions—roots that could be easily overlooked by surgeons who tended to deny the authenticity as well as the conclusions of observations made by persons such as Guy.

Upon inspection of the condition of the blood at the site of the malignancy as compared to elsewhere, Guy went on to speculate that cancer may be caused by a virus that forms in the glands and circulates via the lymphatic system. He asked:

> May it not be reasonably presumed, that the morbid matter of an ulcerated cancer is reabsorbed by those vessels, and by them be carried and lodged in the neighboring glands, and from thence to those more remote?"[7]

He mentions travel from the breast to the axillary glands and demonstrates thereby an understanding of the process whereby spread and metastasis of cancer occur.

It is difficult to read such a work and continue to believe that all medical practices of previous eras were based on mere superstitions. Rather, many protocols may have been based on detailed observations and extensive clinical experience, experience that was carefully handed down to each succeeding generation.

Guy became famous for his nonsurgical treatment of cancer. Though jealous adversaries tried to obtain his secret from him on the grounds that it would serve mankind, Guy did not divulge the Plunkett family's formula. It thus became the object of invective criticism by Guy's chief rival, Thomas Gataker, surgeon to certain members of the British Royal family. Gataker faulted Guy for purchasing a cure from a layman.

To this day we know nothing of Guy's ingredients, but procedures for the nonsurgical removal of tumors were common among American Indians. Even a century before Guy, these techniques were already well-known in both the Colonies and Europe.

CONSTANTINE RAFINESQUE AND SAMUEL THOMSON
Early 1800s

As we have seen, many New World herbalists as well as some surgeons attributed their remedies to Native American medicine men and women who used a wide variety of poultices and pastes to draw cancer out through the skin. Two of the more colorful medical herbalists of these times were Constantine Rafinesque and Samuel Thomson.

Rafinesque was born in Constantinople in 1784 and came to the United States as a young man. He explored the Mississippi Valley, studied the flora, and became well acquainted with the Indians of the region. In 1819 he became a professor of botany and, between 1828 and 1832, he wrote a book called *Medical Flora of the United States* which became the bible of botanic physicians of his day. Rafinesque believed that "There are several modes of effecting cures by equivalent remedies; but vegetable substances afford the mildest, most efficacious and most congenial to the human frame." Among his many contributions to medical botany is an expert description of the medicinal properties of goldenseal, perhaps the most prized of all New World herbs.

Samuel Thomson (1769–1843) was as uneducated as Rafinesque was scholarly. Both men, however, deserve recognition for their accomplishments. Each, in his own way, played a major role in the resurrection of botanical medicine: Rafinesque through his academic appeal to professional physicians and Thomson through his sway over the laity.

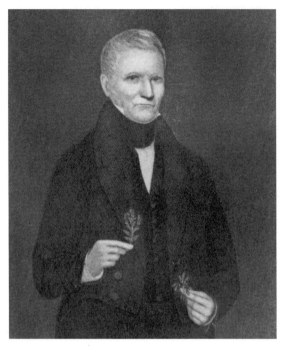

Samuel Thomson, February 9, 1769-October 4, 1843.
SOURCE: *Bulletin of the Lloyd Library,* Reproduction Series, No. 7, frontispiece

Thomson's system of medicine is considered by some experts to be entirely derivative rather than new. His use of emetics, heat producing herbs, and steam are in all likelihood Native American in origin. Thomson believed that illness is caused by cold and relieved by heat. In 1809, Thomson was charged with murder for sweating two children to death and for killing Captain Trickey, a man Thomson claimed never to have treated. He was acquitted and went on, in 1813 and 1823, to obtain patents from the Government for his system of botanic medicine. The patents enabled him to sell rights to his work. In 1822 Thomson published the *New Guide to Health*. He claimed to have sold "family rights," for the then hefty sum of twenty dollars, to 100,000 purchasers. With

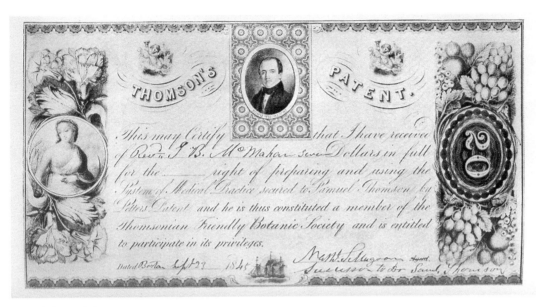

Samuel Thomson's Patent

SOURCE: *Bulletin of the Lloyd Library,* Reproduction Series, No. 7, insert between pages 90-91.

this publication, he set out to take medicine away from the tyranny of the elite and to put it into the hands of the people.

Though Thomson remained controversial, mainly for his touting of lobelia, he is generally credited with the development of a cancer plaster made from red clover blossoms. Though he may have learned about this treatment from the Penobscot Indians, it is likely that he was the first to record the procedures that are still discussed among medical herbalists.

There were tenets to Thomson's system that had wide mass appeal, and Thomson himself was almost a cult leader. By 1839 his followers numbered nearly three million. One detractor referred to him as "one of those illegitimate sons of Æsculapius, who have arisen from time to time to vex the souls of the regular profession." [8]

Thomson's life resembled that of his twentieth century compatriot, Harry Hoxsey: endless confrontations, legal battles, and tireless struggles to gain credibility for his system. He died in Boston in 1843, and historians are still trying to assess his role in medicine. Some view him as the epitome of the Jacksonian Democratic spirit in medicine: a champion for the laboring classes, a challenger of the medical monopoly, and a man of common sense without much schooling. Paul Starr, in his Pulitzer Prize-winning book *The Social Transformation of American Medicine*, states:

> Lay healers in the early nineteenth century saw the medical profession as a bulwark of privilege, and they adopted a position hostile to both its therapeutic tenets and social aspirations. [9]

By the end of the Inquisition (1834), "official" cancer treatment—as two thousand years before—consisted mainly of surgical and caustic treatments. Though Native Americans were apparently conversant with asepsis, Europeans were not. Surgery was therefore conducted under horrific conditions, but the caustic treatments were little better. Justamond, an eighteenth century surgeon, introduced caustic treatments to England. Girouard, another surgeon, advocated adoption of this method in France in 1841. The method used in France involved multiple piercings "in every direction" of the affected area with a sharp, pointed instrument called a trocar. Pure zinc chloride was then poured into the bleeding wounds. The agony, according to John Pattison (1866), was so great that the patient fainted during each operation. The procedure was usually repeated four times.

The purpose behind these barbarous forms of treatment was to destroy (with caustics) or cut away (with the knife) the tumor and its surrounding structure. Because of excessive bleeding, visual inspection of the site was virtually impossible; moreover, recurrence was practically inevitable, occurring in 90 to 99 percent of cases.

These two methods, surgery and caustics, were studied and reported to the French Academy of Science by Dr. Leroy d'Etoilles in 1844. In a report entitled "On the Utility of Surgical Operations in Cancer," the documents of 174 practitioners were analyzed in what was very likely the first five-year survival study of cancer. The French research made comparisons between those who refused treatment and those who were "properly" treated according to the medical precepts of the day.[10] Of the 2,781 patients diagnosed with cancer, many declined treatment of any type. Two-thirds of the persons in the study, 1,873 patients, survived for five years or more. Of these, 1,172 had refused treatment, but it is not known how many of the remaining had surgery and how many were treated using caustics. The protocols used in the caustic treatments are also unknown, although it can be assumed that most involved acids such as nitric acid or sulfuric acid mixed with saffron; poisonous minerals such as lead, mercury, or arsenic nitrate; or alkaline caustics such as sulfate of zinc. Copper sulfate (mixed with borax), quicklime, or potassium permanganate were also sometimes used, evidently with mixed success. In any event, the options of patients in those times were so abhorrent that more patients refused treatment than accepted the procedures that were normal a hundred and fifty years ago.

This statistical effort, though a milestone, was more impressive for its scale than its conclusions. According to the report, after the first five years, those who did not treat their conditions outlived those who underwent the recommended treatments involving surgery or caustics. *Despite the conclusions*, these methods remained standard until the turn of the century when radium (1903) became the new source of hope and promise. Initially, radium was used as an implant in much the same way that the piercings and pouring of caustics had been used. Needles or pellets were implanted directly into tumors until the structure of the malignancy was altered.

Interestingly, an approach similar to that of d'Etoilles was employed as recently as 1990 by Dr. Ulrich Abel, biostatistician of the University of Heidelberg in Germany. Inquiries were sent to oncologists concerning their treatments with cytotoxic drugs (chemotherapy), and the responses of 150 doctors were similarly discouraging. Perhaps we are not winning the "war on cancer" because some of the genuinely effective treatments remain obscure.

In any event, after scrutiny of the findings by d'Etoilles, the time had come for a fresh spirit of inquiry, and the voices came from America to London in the persons of Drs. Fell and Pattison.

Dr. J. Weldon Fell
1858

North American Indians living along the shores of Lake Superior used the red sap from bloodroot to treat cancer.[11]

Based on the unconfirmed reports of traders, Dr. J. Weldon Fell developed a highly successful cancer treatment using bloodroot (*Sanguinaria canadensis*), zinc chloride, flour, and water. Fell coated cotton cloth with the paste, placed it over the tumor, and changed the dressings daily. If the tumor was deep, he used nitric acid to break through healthy tissue. After the tumor began to develop into a slough, he made incisions in the slough, half an inch apart, and inserted the paste into the cuts. This method resulted in the destruction of the tumor and separation of the necrotized mass from the healthy tissue; this usually occurred within ten to fourteen days although sometimes up to four weeks was required.

Fell was on the faculty of New York University and was one of the founders of the New York Academy of Medicine. He moved to London and, in the 1850s, worked at Middlesex Hospital where he conducted cancer treatment studies, primarily of breast cancer patients. Of those patients treated with the bloodroot paste, all showed evidence of remissions of the original growths. Fell's escharotic treatments were successfully compared to surgery. It was learned that eight out of ten surgical patients returned for treatment within two years after their operations, whereas only three out of ten patients treated with the bloodroot paste had a recurrence of cancer within that time.

Fell published his studies in 1858 and, as we shall see, in that same year, another American living in London, John Pattison, published a nearly identical formula using goldenseal (*Hydrastis canadensis*) rather than bloodroot.[12] The addition of zinc chloride to the traditional Native American preparation seems to have originated with Fell who said that this modification allowed for the destruction of large, ulcerated tumors within a few

SLOUGH
A mass of dead tissue that is cast out from living tissue; it can be compared to a scab.

weeks. As we have seen, zinc chloride was already in use by those employing mineral caustics (and the trocar) in their cancer treatments.

Fell's work was carefully reviewed by his peers who concluded that the method was safe, that it could be used on inoperable cancers, and that it spared the patient both the removal of breasts and the dangers of surgery. They noted, too, that enucleation was followed by healthy granulation of the tissues.

Even before Fell introduced bloodroot to his British colleagues, the herb was a popular folk medicine. It was a highly regarded constituent of medicines in both the United States and Russia. Along with the may apple (*Podophyllum peltatum*)—whose use was learned from the Penobscot Indians of Maine—bloodroot was used in the treatment of warts, nasal polyps, and skin cancer. While Fell took his bloodroot cure to England, physicians in Mississippi and Missouri developed treatments using the rhizome of the may apple.

In modern times, experiments with the so-called active ingredients of herbs have proven that the alkaloids in bloodroot (sanguinarine and chelerythrine) have a necrotizing effect on carcinomas and sarcomas of mice. The resin of the may apple (podophyllin) has also been found effective in cancer treatment, particularly ovarian cancer.

Moreover, Fell's work with bloodroot has been replicated with similarly impressive results in recent years by Frederic Mohs, M.D., whose treatment is now standard for basal cell carcinomas and is discussed at the end of this chapter.

ENUCLEATION
The removal of a mass from its supporting tissue. For purposes of this book, enucleation refers to a process that is capable of differentiating healthy from malignant tissue so that the cancerous material separates from normal tissue and then falls away from the body.

GRANULATION
The formation of small, rounded masses in the repair of wounds in soft tissue.

JOHN PATTISON, M.D.
1866

John Pattison was less successful among his peers than his contemporary and fellow American J. Weldon Fell. He, too, had once been affiliated with New York University, but Pattison was more eclectic and holistic than Fell and, perhaps for that very reason, was more difficult to understand. In his 1866 publication, reporting on thirteen years of experience during which he treated over four thousand patients who had cancer, he claimed the "honor" of having been the first to employ *Hydrastis canadensis*, or goldenseal, in the treatment of cancer. Use of hydrastis was learned from the Cherokees. It was introduced to European practitioners in 1760 and gained medical recognition in 1798. Pattison said that goldenseal possesses, "to a certain extent, a specific effect on the disease itself, but has the important advantage of preventing, in a great measure, the pain that would otherwise arise, whilst the destructive power of the zinc is increased." [13]

Pattison called his procedure *enucleation*. He developed great skill in applying his enucleating paste and considered enucleation to be a form of operation because it removed the disease. However, he regarded this procedure as an aid to treatment, not a cure, believing the constitutional remedies—many of them homeopathic—to be more important. As might be expected of someone conversant with homeopathy, he had few hard and fast rules. Treatments were adapted to each patient; and, consequently, the protocols were not particularly subject to memorization, although he described nuances of his procedure and listed many of the remedies he used.

> My prescriptions, however, are mainly confined to the new American vegetable alkaloids, the majority of which I have introduced into this country, and whose efficacy in the treatment not only of cancerous but of other diseases, is acknowledged and corroborated by all who have tried them.[14]

Pattison used equal parts of goldenseal, zinc chloride, flour, and water. When properly mixed, they become mucilaginous. If applied to healthy outer layers of the skin, this paste would be mildly irritating; however, if applied to a deep-seated malignant mass, it would, according to Pattison, do more harm than good. Thus, to enable the paste to act on such parts, he found it necessary to break through the outer layer of skin by using "nitric acid of the specific gravity of 1.35." He compared the pain of this procedure to a blister or a mustard plaster, saying that the pain was bearable and only lasted ten to fifteen minutes.

> Indeed, it is no unfrequent occurrence for delicate and acutely sensitive ladies, to submit to this application in my consulting rooms, and within a quarter of an hour to leave, free from pain and suffering.[15]

After using the diluted nitric acid, the surface appeared whitish. Where the tumor was near the surface, or when it had already ulcerated, the use of a caustic to break through the surface of the skin was unnecessary. Pattison next dressed the area with a salve composed of one part of the enucleating paste and nine parts of calendula ointment. This he described as almost painless because the nerves on the surface were "gradually benumbed and destroyed." He increased the strength of the ointment by degrees until the area was thoroughly deadened. This took five to six days.

> After this I draw perpendicular lines about half an inch apart, and parallel to each other, with the point of my instrument; these scratches never penetrating beyond the deadened structure are never felt by the patient; these I dress with narrow strips of cambric (linen), spread with the undiluted paste. This dressing is only retained for an hour or two, and the same kind of dressings are applied from day to day until the disease is destroyed. As the process advances there is a feeling more of discomfort and uneasiness than of pain; this is owing to the circumstance that as the tumour is destroyed, it becomes heavy; but this discomfort can be readily relieved, by care and ingenuity. This process, however, cannot be carried on without giving rise to some constitutional irritation, evidenced by feverishness, loss of appetite, and sometimes restlessness at night, these symptoms being accompanied by torpidity of the liver and bowels.[16]

Pattison goes on to describe the remedies he used for dealing with the secondary symptoms, including nepenthe[b] for sleep and codeine for pain. Like Fell, he treated many cases of breast cancer, "many hundred cases of malignant disease," and states that he "never had the misfortune to lose a patient during this part of the treatment."[17] Treatment time depended on the size and nature of the tumor, five weeks being the longest time required to destroy the disease.

Only after the tumor was deemed totally destroyed did Pattison remove the strips of cloth on which the paste had been spread. Nothing was done for the next four to five days while the line of demarcation between the healthy and necrotized tissue formed. He found that by dressing the area at that time, the process of separation was retarded, so, with experience, he learned not to interfere at this stage. However, as the mass began to separate, he inserted strips of calico with calendula ointment around the enucleated mass. He changed these dressings only once a day because the discharges at the site helped to soften and assist separation. By the tenth day, he could get a finger between the healthy tissue and separating mass; and at this point, he could remove the strips of calico and begin using cotton wool medicated with the same calendula ointment. The tumor would generally fall off somewhere

between the fourteenth and twenty-first day after the removal of the dressings of enucleating paste. The shortest time for such treatment was twelve days and the longest, thirty-three.

Pattison described many cases, stating that the sloughs usually detach on their own while the patient is sleeping or when the dressings are changed. He mentioned one case in which the entire breast was occupied by a large tumor, and the whole breast fell off, bloodlessly and painlessly, as the patient threw on a shawl before going for a walk. Once the mass detached, the entire area was flat and exposed to view—and bloodless. He never forced the process to go faster, and there was never any blood loss; but the area under the mass was often coated with thick, purulent matter. This he again dressed with calendula ointment and continued to do so until the area was cleansed—always inspecting the site to make sure that no trace of the malignancy remained. If any part of the tumor was still present, he dressed the spot with more enucleating paste (only one percent of his cases required this additional treatment).

If any tendency towards even a minor amount of pain or residual was found, Pattison used other preparations such as goldenseal and honey, a hot water infusion of poke root, or some resin. These varied according to the overall appearance of the site and to how the granulation was progressing. This process often required another three to four weeks after the mass detached. During this stage, he began prophylactic measures, remedies that helped to prevent recurrences.

---

[b] This is probably a sleep inducing herbal concoction. The word *nepenthe* comes from the Greek for *not* and *grief,* a decoction used to induce forgetfulness of sorrows and misfortunes. There is an insect eating plant, *nepenthes distillatoria,* that was used by Native Americans and later by homeopaths in the treatment of smallpox; but the nepenthe referred to by Pattison was probably some form of morphia.

Pattison was sensitive to derogatory remarks about his being a "cancer curer," but he strongly believed that cancer is curable. "I have been able to cure, through the Lord's blessing, by these means. . . I do not refer to cases of yesterday, but to ladies who have been well and have remained well for periods of from eight to twelve to fourteen years." He then described how he thought the homeopathic remedies can reach parts that grosser prescriptions cannot address. Of these, *Hydrastis canadensis* occupied the supreme place in his personal pharmacopoeia. This he administered homeopathically as well as topically in his paste. In chapter 7, the alkaloids and homeopathic remedies used by Pattison are reported. For the present, it is sufficient to note that Pattison developed a remarkable treatment that spared patients the knife, the use of which he vehemently opposed. He quoted Druitt, a leading authority on surgery in the last century:

> *The first and most obvious remedy is extirpating by the knife against which must be alleged the facts, that the removal of one affected part cannot remove the diathesis and that the disease is almost sure to return in the original situation or some other.*
>
> *That the removal of the outward cancer, like the pruning of a tree, sometimes seems to raise the activity of the diathesis, and give increased energy to the morbid growth if produced afterwards. That the entire removal of all affected particles of tissue is often unattainable. That some patients are killed by the operation itself, and that some have died from being operated on for what afterwards proved to be no cancer at all.* [18]

Dr. Eli G. Jones
1911

Eli G. Jones, M.D., Ph.D., graduated from the Eclectic Medical College of Pennsylvania in 1870 and Dartmouth Medical College in 1871. Roy Upton of the American Herbalists Guild informed me that escharotic salves were the treatment of choice of the Eclectic[c] physicians. The Lloyd Library in Cincinnati provided two books by Jones, a homeopath as well as a member of the American Association of Physicians and Surgeons, who had over forty years of experience in the treatment of more than 20,000 cancer patients.

Jones was exceedingly well acquainted with escharotic pastes and regarded them to be local, as opposed to systemic, treatments. In the early part of his career as a cancer specialist, he relied heavily on the pastes. Jones used essentially traditional allopathic caustics combined with bloodroot and sometimes galangal or red saunders (sandalwood). As such, he was a bridge between the naturopathic practitioners and medical professionals of his day.

DIATHESIS
Predisposition to a particular disease.

---

[c] The term *eclectic* was first used by Constantine S. Rafinesque (1784-1841) to describe those who *adopt in practice whatever is found beneficial*. The Eclectic Medical Institute was founded by Wooster Beach (1794-1868) in the 1830s as an alternative to the bloodletting that was standard in his times.

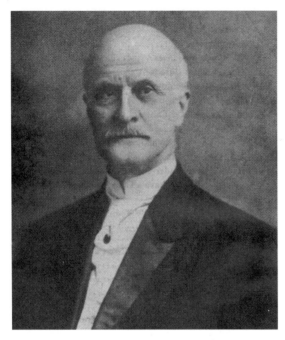

Dr. Eli G. Jones
SOURCE: *Cancer: Its Causes Symptoms & Treatment*, page 6

Jones was one more link in a chain dating back to the Father of modern medicine, Hippocrates. Unlike Guy and the Plunkett family with their secret formula, it was Americans like Fell, Pattison, and Jones who lifted the veil of secrecy that had historically surrounded the use of salves and other botanic remedies used to treat cancer. Jones began offering training seminars in 1894. In 1905 and 1911,[19] he published detailed accounts of his protocols for different types of cancer. He further differed from nearly all of his predecessors by referring to those who relied exclusively on escharotics as quacks, his logic being that cancer is a constitutional condition affecting the blood so it must be treated internally as well as externally.

There is no plaster, caustic or salve that can be applied to a Cancer that will cure it without internal treatment for the blood.[20]

It is not clear where the idea that cancer is a disease of the blood originated. We note that Richard Guy did examine the blood at the site of the tumor, but the belief was more widely held on the American side of the Atlantic than in the Old World. Iroquois medicine men thought cancer to be systemic, a poison that corrupts the body as a result of poor dietary choices, such as foods that cause too much acidity in the body. Cancer then erupts wherever the tissue is tender. They prescribed pipsissewa, *Chimaphila umbellata*, for the stomach.[d]

In the chronology of salve use, very few professional practitioners combined escharotic treatments with internal tonics. However, as previously noted, Hildegard had a duckweed elixir and yarrow brew that she felt reduced the risk of metastases. Examination of lay manuals suggests that alteratives (blood purifiers) were, in fact, widely used by Indian medicine men and women and their followers. The most famous of these came to be known as *trifolium compound*, a tonic made of red clover blossoms and a number of other common American herbs. It was used by Eclectic physicians, medicine men, and lay practitioners—and it is still widely available today. Pattison and Jones were among the first professional physicians to emphasize the need for combining external treatments with internal ones.

[d] See appendix B, page 189.

Jones was an assiduous student, and after many years of "constant study," he, like Pattison, concluded that the internal remedies were more important than the pastes. He maintained that the reason so many doctors failed to cure cancer was that they ignored the systemic nature of the disease and did not employ internal cures. Nevertheless, he published four escharotic formulae that he found to be effective as well as the formulae for various poultices and a yellow healing salve. The cornerstone of his protocol was, however, *scrophularia compound*, a syrup with figwort that seems quite worthy of further investigation. [21]

Jones saw more cases of breast cancer (4,300 cases, including 100 men) than any other form of cancer, and he differentiated a number of types of breast cancer. The largest tumor he ever removed using escharotic treatments was twenty-two inches in circumference and weighed four and one-half pounds. Jones used his Paste No.1[22] for six days, then the poultice, then the healing salve. The woman was cured of cancer but died of heart disease three years later.

By the turn of the century, escharotic pastes were apparently available in virtually every corner drug store in the United States, much as aspirin is today. My sources indicate that they are still widely available in the Carolinas, Tennessee, Oklahoma, Colorado, Wyoming, Montana, the Dakotas, Nevada, and Utah. That the popular use of the salves is today more widespread among lay practitioners than health care professionals in no way affects the efficacy of the treatment method—merely its proper understanding and availabil-

ity. Hopefully, this book will promote a deeper appreciation and insight into a neglected method of cancer treatment, this by physicians as well as holistic health care professionals and their patients.

JOHANNA BRANDT
1928

Johanna Brandt, in her book *The Grape Cure*, copyrighted in 1928, reported that "In South Africa, many people 'draw out' cancer with herbal poultices. They have had great results in some cases. The wound caused by this process becomes a sort of *safety-valve* through which so much poison is eliminated that the patient is saved from an immediate recurrence of the disease."[23] Her view was presented in such an impartial manner as to warrant the respect of even some critics.

We see, nonetheless, that the risk of recurrence has been observed and factored into treatment considerations for centuries. Even in the twelfth century, Hildegard of Bingen suggested the use of yarrow to prevent metastasis. Speculations as to how and why metastasis occurs may differ from era to era and between different schools of medical thought, but the danger has been recognized for at least two thousand years. Therefore, however devoted to their remedies they were, the exponents of external herbal applications only compared their use to surgery, not to anything regarded as more constitutional, regenerative, or preventative in action.

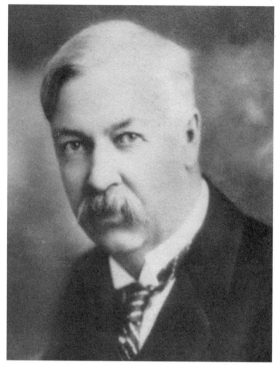

Dr. Perry Nichols
SOURCE: *The Value of Escharotics*

PERRY NICHOLS, M.D.
1929 and 1934

For many years, Dr. Perry Nichols operated a respected and successful sanatorium for the treatment of cancer. Like many of his predecessors, he did not divulge his escharotic formula. Rather, he published a handsome annual, a book consisting mainly of testimonials by satisfied patients. One has the sense that discharged patients felt themselves to be members of a club of persons fortunate enough to have heard of the Nichols Sanatorium and to have had treatment there before submitting to loss of body parts and radium implants, the fashion of the day.

On the basis of the testimony of patients, several of whom were themselves physicians, Nichols appears to have had success rivaling Dr. John Pattison and Dr. Eli Jones. However, he did not believe that cancer has anything to do with the condition of the blood or that internal tonics were necessary. He relied exclusively on escharotic treatments, poultices, and eventual skin grafting to deal with the scars resulting from the salve treatments.

Nichols did train other physicians. He said that regardless of their prior background, it took four years to become proficient in the application of his escharotic treatment. Those who attempt such cures without proper training were, in his opinion, quacks. The techniques used at the Nichols Sanatorium do not seem to have been preserved nearly as well as his annual publications. Nichols described his escharotic as a "double compound," four times the strength of chloride of zinc plaster or arsenical (Marsden) paste. Whatever his compound, he stated that it would destroy any living tissue. Nichols therefore used it so as to destroy the tumor plus a margin around the tumor. He removed the eschar with a curette. The site was then poulticed. In contrast to Pattison, Nichols believed that the stronger escharotics were safer and more effective. He compared his method to a sharp surgical knife:

> *That which is most rapid is the best, because some cancers will grow faster than a slow treatment can kill them . . . Strange as it may at first seem, that which will act with the greatest rapidity is the least painful. You are well aware that a sharp*

*knife will cut deeply into the flesh, with but
little irritation or pain, and yet do but little cutting. So it is with escharotics. The
strong, penetrating will do more in a
shorter time, and with less pain, than the
slow or irritating one.*[24]

Nichols quotes liberally from the professional journals of his day. He refers to specialists at the Mayo Clinic and Johns Hopkins who
acknowledged the superiority of caustics over
surgery. An excerpt from *The Annals of Surgery*,
July 1907, from an article by William Stuart
Halstead, surgeon at Johns Hopkins, makes a
point: "I have several times had occasion to
operate upon cancer which had been vigorously and repeatedly treated with caustics
(escharotics) and to note the comparatively
admirable conditions, the freedom from cancer
permeation of the surrounding tissues and of
the axilla; whereas, after incomplete operation
with the knife, the local manifestations of
recurrence were almost invariably deplorable,
and the prognosis, of course, invariably hopeless."

Nichols treated 19,000 patients over the
course of more than thirty years. He turned
away those he was certain he could not cure.
These included cases of people on their last
legs with metastatic conditions as well as cancers of the stomach, uterus, and liver. Of the
others, he described some who arrived with
but little chance of cure and some who were
properly treated in the early stages of the disease. He said the prognosis was about 50 percent for those whose conditions were advanced
and 90 percent for the others. Overall, of

those accepted for treatment, his cure rate was
75 percent.

HARRY HOXSEY
1901–1974

Harry Hoxsey looked the part of a classic
snake oil salesman. He completed high school
by correspondence course; and, though aspir-
ing to be a doctor, he never went to college.
He began treating patients while merely a
youngster and eventually had a chain of cancer
clinics, staffed by properly trained and licensed
medical doctors, spreading throughout seven-
teen states.

Hoxsey used an internal tonic, popularly
called *Elixirex*, that he claimed his great-grandfather had developed in 1840 after watching a
horse cure itself of cancer by grazing on herbs.
This sounds a bit fanciful. There may have been
a horse, even a horse with cancer who foraged
in a meadow, but not on potassium iodide (one
of the ingredients of the tonic). It is more
likely that Hoxsey's tonic[e] is but one of the
many variations of a traditional red clover tonic
used for centuries.

In any event, Hoxsey obtained his internal
cancer formula from his father who got it from
his father who got it from his father—another
family secret passed on for generations.
Hoxsey also used trichloroacetic acid; a red
external salve containing bloodroot, zinc chloride, and antimony sulfide; and a yellow heal-

---

[e] The formula for *Elixirex* is in appendix B, page 195.

ing powder made of sublimed sulfur, arsenic trisulfide, elder blossoms, and magnolia flowers. Whatever the history of the Hoxsey protocol, the paste is but one in a steady stream of escharotic formulae with their accompanying internal cancer tonics.

Despite the fact that Hoxsey himself did not technically treat patients in his clinics, he was arrested more times than anyone else in medical history, usually on charges of practicing medicine without a license. Throughout his career, Hoxsey was surrounded by patients and doctors who were convinced that his treatment was superior to any other in use at the time. Many of these people testified in court on his behalf, and he was acquitted in a number of trials. However, all testimony was based on personal experience and the medical expertise of individual doctors rather than on "science."

Hoxsey was indefatigable. He forever challenged the American Medical Association (AMA), state medical institutions, and the Federal Government to conduct a proper investigation of his treatments. Uncompromising and inflexible, he put forth terms proposing that skeptics select any one hundred subjects out of a group of patients having proper pathological proofs of cancer. Hoxsey would have these patients treated free of charge and would guarantee that they would be cancer free in twelve weeks with no recurrences within five years. If 80 percent of the patients responded in this way, the Hoxsey protocol would be entitled to a proper medical review; if he failed to deliver the results, they could brand him a quack. Hoxsey steadfastly

refused to divulge the contents of his formulae, declaring that he would do so only after tests were conducted. The AMA, National Cancer Institute (NCI), and other organizations never agreed to his conditions.

> *The method of treatment must be explained fully. There must be no secrecy whatsoever in regard to the composition or nature of the treatment.* [25]

Hoxsey eventually gave in, but the NCI faulted his submissions and closed the matter. Over the years, numerous competent investigators testified that Hoxsey's methods were remarkably successful, but Hoxsey never gained medical sanction for his treatments— partly, no doubt, because of a curious belief that only people with proper credentials can cure illness. Scoffers insist, for example, that a horse cannot develop a cancer cure. This mind set is best exemplified by the oft quoted statement of William Grigg, Public Information Officer of the FDA:

> *The idea that the American Indians, or this person or that person . . . would accidentally stumble upon some herb that would cure (cancer) is rather far-fetched. It's like the idea that if you put three billion monkeys in a room, one of them might write a Shakespearean sonnet.* [26]

Nevertheless, there is a new field of herbalism called "zoopharmacognosy" based on observations of animals who medicate themselves naturally and "who practice medicine without a license." There is also considerable interest in the medicinal properties of herbs that might be useful in treating illness. For instance, researchers would like to know what Amazonians use to shrink heads because the same substances might be useful in reducing the size of tumors.

Hoxsey was not to benefit by these modern queries. In 1953, the United States Senate-commissioned FitzGerald Report concluded that organized medicine had conspired to suppress the Hoxsey treatments as well as many other therapies. A year later, a team of ten medical doctors, after spending two days at Hoxsey's Dallas clinic, signed a unanimous declaration stating that the clinic was successfully treating "pathologically proven cases of cancer, both internal and external." [27] His remedies had become the foremost cancer treatment in the United States, but they had not achieved official approval. Eventually, continuous harassment forced Hoxsey to move his work to Tijuana, Mexico, in 1963.

There was no question as to whether or not Hoxsey's formulae worked: a Federal court in Dallas ruled that the Hoxsey treatments were comparable in effectiveness to surgery, chemotherapy, and x-ray. The issue was economic. Even the AMA, which at one time tried to buy patents for the internal tonic from Hoxsey and which later became the agent of the relentless persecution of Hoxsey, eventually admitted that the external salve had merit. As recently as 1990, the primary criticism of the external treatment was that it was "archaic." [28]

The elixir's anticancer potential was officially acknowledged in a paper prepared for the U.S. Congress's Office of Technology Assessment by Patricia Spain Ward who researched the therapeutic benefit of the individual herbs in the formula. "Orthodox scientific research has by now identified antitumor activity" in most of the plants used in the Hoxsey internal tonic. Although not every herb in the tonic was deemed capable of inhibiting malignancy, the synergy of the entire formula has never been researched, nor has the possible immune-boosting effect of the herbs been studied.

With the paste, the conclusions are, however, clear: it has been found to be effective in the treatment of cancer by scores of investigators over several centuries.[f]

Dr. John Christopher
1909–1983

Dr. John Christopher was a naturopathic doctor living in Utah. Persecuted for healing, he became a teacher, lecturer, and prolific writer. Christopher's cancer protocols were summarized in *The Layman's Course on Killing Cancer* by Sam Biser and later revised and reissued by his brother, Loren Biser,[29] both students of Christopher's. *The Layman's Course* is not only a fascinating compilation of treatments but also the latest in a tradition of

---

[f] The Hoxsey formulae are given in appendix B.

botanical publications for lay use going back several hundred years. Elements of Christopher's work, as well as his confrontations with the law, resemble those of Samuel Thomson who died in 1843.

Formulae for two pastes used by Christopher in the treatment of cancer are described by the Bisers. They reported that some patients experienced a complete regression of tumors in one week, while the treatment for others had to be continued for two months. In the course, the salves are referred to as Red Sun Balm and German Kermesberro.[30]

> To cure[g] skin cancer, you should use the German Kermesberro paste with another mixture called Red Sun Balm. The Red Sun Balm increases the circulation in the area. The German Kermesberro paste draws out the toxins. Together they work very effectively.[31]

Kermesberro, commonly known as poke root (*Phytolacca decandra*), is also sometimes called pigeon berry or inkberry because people in the Southern United States use the berry of the plant for making purple ink. Red Sun Balm is an escharotic using cayenne.

Dr. John Pattison and Dr. Eli Jones, both physicians, and Dr. John Christopher, a naturopath, all had extensive clinical experience in the treatment of persons with cancer. Despite considerable variations in their protocols, they were highly successful in treating a disease that is all too often regarded as incurable by even the most eminent authorities. All three used escharotic treatments in conjunction with internal herbal tonics, tinctures, and teas. What is also perfectly clear is that many of their methods were what might be called "traditional." The techniques were known and respected by their predecessors but developed to very high levels of effectiveness by these practitioners. These doctors should therefore be viewed as outstanding exponents of a system of cure that had been well established for centuries rather than as inventors of the approaches they perfected.

BLACK AND YELLOW SALVES
Current

Professional use of escharotic pastes continues side by side lay use even today. In her book *What Your Doctor Won't Tell You*, Jane Heimlich reports that the late H. Ray Evers, M.D., substantiated some of the claims made for the black and yellow salves, having said that they are beneficial for skin cancers and breast tumors. Evers was director of the International Medical Center in Juarez, Mexico. He died in 1990 and has been succeeded in his work by Dr. Francisco Soto.

Heimlich quotes Ken Michaelis, whose family operated a pharmacy dispensing escharotic preparations, as saying:

> Black and yellow salves, used alternately, open a hole in the flesh and draw out the tumor.[32]

---

[g] The word *cure* has been retained in order to remain faithful to the original text. However, it remains to be determined whether or not escharotic pastes are, in fact, a cure for cancer, or rather a treatment that is best combined with other therapies.

The formulae for these particular black and yellow salves, like many of the historic salves, were passed down through several generations to the woman who makes them today. She told me that when her husband developed liver cancer in 1977, she made up the salves. He used them for a time in 1977 and 1978, and he is alive as of this writing.

When I first heard about the salves, I called Ken Michaelis to find out more about them. He supplied a large number of anecdotal accounts, but nothing subject to verification. I asked him to refer me to a practitioner experienced in the use of the products. He gave me the name of a medical doctor whom I contacted and who claimed to have treated 10,000 patients without a single complication or death attributable to salve use. His emphasis was on the incredible safety of the method.

Recently, one of my students who had cancer a number of years ago went to a clinic specializing in long-term detoxification. She said that they were using black and yellow "patches" that seemed similar to the salves described in this book. There are today a number of such "black salves," often used in conjunction with yellow healing ointments. There are also several variations of something called "Compound X," formulae that resemble the black salves except that they are generally used as stand-alone preparations, i.e. without poultices or healing salves.

FREDERIC E. MOHS, M.D.
1910–

Our last story brings us to the present time. Frederic Mohs, M.D., of the University of Wisconsin, did extensive research with what he called a *fixative paste*, an external preparation containing bloodroot, zinc chloride, and stibnite (an ore of antimony consisting mainly of antimony trisulfide).[33] Mohs claimed that by having granules of different sizes, he could control the tissue penetration of zinc chloride, a substance he first used in animal experiments as an irritant injected into transplanted cancers. Upon sectioning the tissues, he discovered that the microscopic features of the killed tissues were well-preserved, i.e., fixed.

Mohs came to realize that he could remove malignancies with complete microscopic control if the borders between the neoplasms and normal tissue were clearly demarcated. It seems that, through trial and error, he developed an enucleating plaster without realizing exactly what other functions the paste performed.

In his vast bibliography, no mention is made of his predecessors in the nineteenth century. Mohs gives an account of the process whereby he arrived at his ultimate formula, but my sense is that "of the many organic materials tested," it was no accident that he ended up with bloodroot "to prevent the zinc chloride from settling to the bottom of the container."

Mohs developed a technique called *chemosurgery* that may be the bridge between traditional escharotic treatments of cancer and modern surgery. In the Mohs method, the fixative paste is applied to visible and palpable tumors to facilitate clear demarcation between the malignant and healthy tissue. To "produce fixation *in situ*," the paste is applied some hours or days before surgical excision of chemically fixed tissue, the undersurface of which is microscopically scanned. This is a technical way of saying that by looking underneath the tissue that is surgically cut away, it can be determined by the margins whether or not all the malignancy has been removed. What seems equally important is that after removing the visible cancer, another layer of paste is applied to the open wound. The site is bandaged and checked again, usually in twenty-four hours. The process is repeated, sometimes daily over the course of two weeks, until the margins of the removed tissue are clear. The final step in the Mohs technique is another application of the paste. Since this last step is not for the purpose of demarcating malignant tissue, it is evidently a safety precaution aimed at the destruction of whatever remains of the tumors.

The Mohs method is used on many types of cancer, and its effectiveness has been studied on tens of thousands of patients. In the 1960s, various teams of doctors reported the complete healing of cancers of the nose, external ear, and other organs using a paste of bloodroot and zinc chloride.[34] Ralph W. Moss, Ph.D., former assistant director of public affairs at Memorial Sloan-Kettering Cancer Center, quoted an Office of Technology Assessment report (1990) stating that Mohs achieved 99 percent success for all primary basal cell carcinomas he treated—the highest success rate reported for any method of cancer treatment.[35] The Mohs treatment, though not often used for deeper tumors, is now standard for certain forms of skin cancer.

Dr. Mohs was not available to discuss his treatment, so I spoke with Dr. Stephen Snow, one of the physicians who took over the practice of Dr. Mohs when he retired. Snow exhibited a fascinating familiarity with microscopy. He described cancerous cells as linked "like brothers and sisters holding hands." Part of the advantage of microscopic examination is that physicians are enabled to track the malignancy to the end of the chain. What one sees on the surface is like the tip of an iceberg, but microsurgery allows the surgeon to focus on what remains beneath the normal view. Snow also described the escharotic treatment as a kind of "heat sink" that creates "regional hyperthermia" that constitutes a kind of "scorched earth" approach to cancer destruction. Since water is the main constituent of the body, this approach is only effective if the heat manages to pass through the insulating barrier of moisture.

Snow continued by saying that most people understand what they see, but not what they do not see, and that there remains much to be learned about cellular biology. Snow felt that the Mohs method constitutes a softer way of looking at cancer and its treatment, but presenting this understanding to his peers is a concern. As an example, he felt that the paste might have an immunologic effect as well as escharotic action, but this dimension of the treatment has never been fully researched.

Further, Snow commented that in this day of instant gratification, cancer patients often want their conditions cured immediately. As such, the method is not as popular as might be expected, for even with basal and squamous cell carcinomas and melanomas, the Mohs technique requires at least twenty-four hours—and the patient wants to shorten this to two. If this is a problem with skin cancers, imagine the challenge of deeper malignancies such as occur in the breast.

As the final version of this book was being edited prior to going to press, there was a report on Cable News Network (CNN) that to reduce medical costs, "drive through mastectomies" were to replace the hospitalization currently normal for such major procedures. Personally, I am still in shock. It is obviously important for surgeons and patients to assess the pros and cons of surgical removal of tumors versus some less drastic treatment that would make it possible to save a breast—or some other organ. Where cancer is concerned, surgery is neither a panacea nor an instant solution. Recovery often takes months and may never be complete, especially if followed by edema, various efforts at reconstructive surgery, and partial loss of function. Besides, surgery in no way guarantees that cancer will not recur. Therefore, if efficiency is offered as a medical justification for why cancer is being treated as it is today, it is probably because patients do not really understand that they have choices—and they realize too late what recovery entails.

SUMMARY OF ESCHAROTIC HISTORY

Cancer treatment today remains a matter of great controversy. Surgery is perhaps the most effective of the three standard cancer treatments (surgery, chemotherapy, and radiation), but the cure rate is as disappointing as centuries earlier. Salves have been promoted by some as a cure-all. Responsible practitioners, lay and professional alike, have steadfastly maintained that escharotics are merely an alternative to surgery and that they may offer an alternative to the loss of body parts and the complications that arise when the body is no longer whole. Some regard the salves as a kind of botanical surgeon. Others, because of the fact that some of the salve is absorbed into the blood stream and because a heat reaction accompanies their use, see escharotics as a mixture of surgery, chemotherapy, and even radiation.

Modern surgery is no longer as dangerous as it was even fifty years ago, not to mention earlier. However, even if it is less primitive, many contemporary cancer protocols are not really less tortuous than centuries ago. Compared to surgery and chemotherapy, escharotic cancer treatments are both less invasive and less painful. However, the salves are not fun to use, neither do they offer assurance that death can be forestalled. Nevertheless, they are an option; and, when used correctly, their effectiveness has been continuously demonstrated by each succeeding generation.

Summary of Various Escharotic Methods

500 B.C.	Ancient India	Arsenic paste
460-377 B.C.	Hippocrates	Caustics and cautery
12th century	Hildegard of Bingen	Violet salve with duckweed elixir and yarrow anti-metastasis beverage
16th century	Fallopius	Caustics
	Penobscot Indians	Bloodroot and/or may apple poultices and plasters
17th century	Scores of papers	Herbal poultices, plasters, ointments
1759	Richard Guy	Enucleating plaster
1769-1843	Samuel Thomson	*New Guide to Health*, 1822, family rights; red clover blossom paste and black salve
1784-1841	Constantine Rafinesque	Reports on Indian medicines, *Medical Flora*, 1828-32
1844	Dr. Leroy-d'Etoilles French Academy of Science	Five-year survival study based on surgery, caustics, and refusal of treatment
1855	Daniel Smith	Red onion and bloodroot powder; poke root, jimson seeds, boar's tusk root; pipsissewa tea
1858	Dr. J. Weldon Fell	Bloodroot and zinc chloride paste with incisions in eschar, peer review
1866	Dr. John Pattison	Goldenseal enucleating paste and calendula ointment, herbal alkaloids, and homeopathic remedies
1904	William Fox, M.D.	Blue flag, red clover, bloodroot tinctures
1911	Dr. Eli G. Jones	Bloodroot or poke root escharotics, followed by poultices and/or homeopathic remedies, tinctures, oils; healing salve; scrophularia compound (tonic for internal use.)
1928	Johanna Brandt, N.D.	Grape cure; safety-valve
1929	Perry Nichols, M.D.	Escharotic with curette and plastic surgery; no internal treatment
died 1974	Harry Hoxsey	Trichloroacetic acid; escharotic made of antimony, blood root, and zinc chloride; yellow powder containing sulfur; internal red clover combination tonic
died 1983	Dr. John Christopher	Cayenne salve and poke root healing ointment; many teas; internal tonics including red clover combination formula; herbal bolus
died 1990	H. Ray Evers, M.D.	Black escharotic and yellow healing salve
born 1910	Frederic E. Mohs, M.D.	Antimony, bloodroot, and zinc chloride paste; microsurgery technique published in 1956 and 1978

CHAPTER 2

Types of Cancer Salves

Since there are a wide variety of cancer salves, it may be useful to begin with a survey of their types, historic to the present. As noted in chapter 1, the most popular of the salves are what are called escharotic pastes. *Webster's Dictionary* says that escharotic means "scar forming." However, most practitioners using the term are referring to a caustic substance that is capable of producing a *slough*, a mass of dead tissue that eventually separates from the living tissue and falls away from the body. Escharotic preparations may be acid or base. They may be made of minerals or acids or herbs or some mixture of chemical and botanical ingredients.

I have differentiated three basic types of herbal cancer salves: (1) those that destroy the tumor by causing a chemical reaction that gives rise to heat; (2) those that act more directly on the tumor by necrotizing the tumor on contact; a "chemical" reaction, but not necessarily one producing heat; and (3) those that stimulate circulation, perhaps in such a manner as to permit oxygenation of the tissues that are capable of life and thus promote some sort of separation of these healthy tissues from the malignant ones. I feel that by attempting to make such differentiations, I may be guilty of splitting hairs; but the salves are not all the same even though many of them combine characteristics of all three of these categories.

ESCHAROTIC METHOD USING A SINGLE SALVE

So far as I can determine, many practitioners, both lay and professional, used a single escharotic salve, one not supported by any type of external follow-up applications. Historically, Hildegard's salve appeared to be such a salve. The mysterious poultice formula that the eighteenth century surgeon Richard Guy purchased from the Plunkett family might also have been a sort of stand-alone product as was the escharotic used by Dr. J. Weldon Fell. Native American medicine men and lay practitioners who used a tar-like paste made of red clover blossoms also used a single compound—as opposed to a series of different salves depending on the tumor and stage of the process. These formulations were probably used not only for all types of cancers but also for ulcerations of the skin, warts, moles, and localized infections, such as those stemming from wounds or venomous bites. The various contemporary Compound X formulae are such preparations as is the Mohs fixative paste.

Since many salve producers state in their literature that a single application of one paste is sufficient to destroy an entire tumor—a statement that, according to my experience, is probably only true of rather small skin tumors—I feel that this procedure and the assumptions underlying it need to be understood within the context of how escharotics work.

> *Simply stated, if the salve does not penetrate the entire tumor, no matter what the salve contains and what the theory behind it is, the tumor will not be completely destroyed. Thus, even if a dramatic reaction follows use of the salve, it does not necessarily mean that the process is complete.*

Fell and Mohs combined surgical techniques with use of their escharotics. In Fell's technique, incisions were made in the eschar. Paste was inserted into the slits so that the escharotic would penetrate further. Fell was probably the first to modify the bloodroot formula and escharotic technique so as to combine what he, in his day, regarded as the best of botanical med-

NECROTIZE
Death of tissue, usually by injury or disease, but in this usage by escharotic or other action of the herbs.

icine with chemical medicine and surgery. He added zinc chloride to the traditional Native American formula to promote deeper penetration.

With the Mohs method, the eschar is sliced off and examined under a microscope to see if the margins of the tumor are clear. If they are not clear, the process is repeated until there is no further evidence of malignancy. When no surgery is used, there has to be another way to assure that the entire malignancy is necrotized.

At this juncture, I have spent eight years investigating this treatment. All too often I have met with sincere but naïve assumptions regarding the miraculous potentials of the salves. Even if we accept that Hildegard's salve resulted in death of the tumor by contact, we have to realize that in order for the destruction to occur, contact with the tumor has to take place. When the tumor is very large or very deep, it is likely that many applications of a considerable amount of the escharotic will be needed to necrotize the tumor completely. It is also wise to keep in mind that for centuries many practitioners used internal tonics to address whatever the escharotic failed to destroy. Moreover, many of them came to prefer the internal treatments to the external.

SALVES VERSUS PASTES

Hildegard had a genuine salve. Besides the juice of the crushed violets, her preparation contained olive oil and billy goat tallow. Ointments or salves are used because of the capacity of oils to penetrate and carry the botanicals deeper into the tissues. However, many escharotics are water-based pastes, not salves, and they do not penetrate as far as is often assumed.

Zinc chloride, used by many in their otherwise botanical preparations for the last 150 years, can act as a carrier for the other ingredients, but it is not as deeply penetrating as a cerate. Moreover, unless constituting a very small percentage of the total formula, zinc chloride can be excruciatingly painful. While exceptionally sterile, zinc chloride is a caustic that is for all intents and purposes indiscriminately destructive. This is an important point to emphasize since many producers maintain that their products can be used internally as well as externally. In my opinion, zinc chloride is contraindicated for internal use. Aside from its anti-infective properties, it has no constituents or actions that resemble the botanical ingredients in the pastes. It does not restore health or regenerate tissue; it is merely a very potent chemical agent that burns through tissue— though it does to some extent, according to Mohs, have a somewhat greater affinity for malignant than healthy tissue.

Since these issues are covered more later, what should be emphasized at this point is that a single application of an escharotic paste may indeed necrotize a small basal cell carcinoma. However, to do so, the paste must be applied thickly enough to coat the entire mass, and it must be kept occlusive so that the paste does not dry out. If the tumor is deep, large, and not very absorbent, a single application will seldom be adequate. This in no way implies that salve use has to be combined with surgery, merely that blind faith in miraculous possibilities needs to be tempered by a large amount of common sense.

> *Misconceptions can be fatal. In order to obtain the desired results, the potency, correct use, and limitations of whatever product is used need to be properly understood. Moreover, in nearly every instance, bloodroot escharotics need to be used more aggressively than their makers suggest.*

REACTIONS

Various procedures for using escharotics are discussed in chapters 7-9. For the moment, suffice it to say that if the suspected neoplasm reacts with the salve, there will usually be, *at minimum*, an increase in circulation and heat at the application site; often an itchy or burning sensation; and sometimes a greater or lesser amount of pain. Since responses are inconsistent from person to person, from application to application, and from product to product, predictions as to how a given person will react to a particular application are impossible.

CERATE
A substance for external use that is made with an oil or wax or both.

NEOPLASM
A mass of tumorous material.

OCCLUSIVE
"Closed," i.e., air tight.

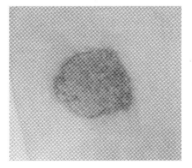

Reaction to an escharotic salve applied on a woman following surgery for ovarian cancer and exceedingly high CA-125 test results.

Depending on the product used and the type of growth, there may or may not be a reaction. If there is a reaction, the surface of the skin will redden; blister; and then turn whitish, grayish, yellowish, greenish-gray, or black. If the application site blisters, there may be anything from tiny pinhead size eruptions to entire areas that change color and texture. This is the beginning of the formation of the eschar or slough. After some days, the eschar will thicken. Later it will begin to crack around the edges. Then, for some days, the eschar may be loose and seem to be hanging on by a thread. Movement at this stage may be uncomfortable, and jostling can sometimes result in a small amount of bleeding. Eventually, the eschar will detach and fall away, usually onto the bandage. This should be allowed to occur naturally without picking or provocation. A "crater" and pinkish new skin, similar to the tissue seen after a scab falls off on its own, plus whatever remains of the tumor will then be visible.

A small skin tumor may fall off in a few days; a larger slough may take ten to twelve days or even longer to detach completely. In the interim, there is usually discharge from the crack around the eschar. The area may weep clear fluids, pus, or other morbid looking matter, often greenish-gray in color with a quite noxious odor. This stage of the treatment may last as little as a day or two or as long as 14–16 days—or longer if using a method involving multiple products. For the patient, the process is generally nothing short of fascinating. However, no matter what the temptations are to peek underneath to see what is happening,

this is not advisable because movement may cause unnecessary pain as well as a little bleeding.

Once the slough has fallen off, a crater will be visible. It is usually very pink and clean looking, sometimes almost flat and sometimes quite deep.[h] The site will be entirely bloodless unless the slough was pulled off prematurely, in which case it will bleed just as a scab might if removed before it comes off on its own. At this point, a careful observer will often be able to see whether any malignancy remains in the treatment area. For an inexperienced person, this sort of judgment is virtually impossible. Basically, what one is looking for is any trace of residual tumor. The chances of destroying the entire malignancy in a single course of escharotic use depends a great deal on the size and location of the tumor as well as the product and method used.

If thin layers of paste were used, the odds of some malignancy remaining in the crater are significant. This is also true when the original mass was large and/or deep. The top of the residual tumor will generally be visible in the crater. This indicates that only the part of the tumor closest to the surface of the skin was necrotized; the rest of the growth remains in the treatment site—and depending on many factors, its growth may have been arrested—or it may have been stimulated by the trauma. At this juncture, careful inspection, a trained eye, and good judgment are needed. Moreover, it is important that the hole not be permitted to

---

[h] Detailed pictures of this process are found in the color section.

close until all malignancy has been removed and all discharges have ceased.

Discharges are common during the entire escharotic process, but they tend to increase as the cracking around the edge progresses. Once the eschar has detached, a small hole in the crater usually becomes visible. Discharges of morbid matter from this hole sometimes continue for weeks or months.

NEXT STEPS

With the single salve approach, there is no other treatment. Application of the salve is simply followed by waiting. It is my guess that such salves are fragments of a more comprehensive procedure whose details have been lost. That the process works for some people is undeniable; that it is safe for everyone seems questionable.

There are those who reapply the escharotic immediately after the first slough falls off, in which case the process involves repetition of essentially the same steps and developments though reactions tend to occur faster. There are also those who recommend waiting a few months or a year before reapplying the salve. Experts, from Pattison through Jones, would no doubt take vehement exception to the notion that it is safe to leave a malignancy in place with the intention of dealing with it later, most especially once blood circulation to the area has been increased and the site itself has

been irritated by treatment. Since many salve producers are convinced to the contrary, it seems appropriate to stress that this opinion belongs to a lay rather than professional tradition of practitioners of this method. It is difficult to argue with those who claim to be heir to the wisdom of generations of salve use; but professional physicians who used the salve on tens of thousands of people over the last two and a half centuries would, while defending the efficacy of nonsurgical treatments of cancer, have valiantly refuted the notion that use of escharotics can be safely suspended for some months while the patient builds up the resolve to continue the treatment. Such statements should probably be regarded as ignorant and dangerous.

DRAWING SALVES

Throughout history and into the present time, more practitioners used a dual salve procedure with, as one might by now expect, considerable variations. The second salve may be either a drawing or a healing salve. Drawing salves usually have some form of tallow as an ingredient.

Though Hildegard—who had a single salve technique—put billy goat tallow in her violet salve compound, tallow is generally only found in the preparations used after the eschar has formed. Drawing salves act just as their name suggests: they pull morbid matter from the opening created by the escharotic salve. This gives rise to a tugging sensation. The following account describes the action of drawing salves:

While in her early thirties, a young mother of two discovered that she had cancer of the left breast. She had a modified radical mastectomy and six months of chemotherapy. Eighteen months later, she learned that she had cervical cancer. Less than two years after the second operation, she was informed that the cancer had metastasized to her liver. She told me that the Bible taught her about food and herbs. She applied the salve over her liver and said that some time later, she felt a jerking sensation in her chest where the breast had been. She said, "I just knew they didn't get it all. It's all traveling down and coming out the hole over my liver."

As she described this and her little almond-shaped hole over the liver to me over the telephone, the excitement she felt was quite moving. This woman did not survive the complications of allopathic intervention (morphine to control gastric distress following injudicious consumption of foods she was unable to digest.) An autopsy revealed no residual of the cancer; but she, unfortunately, did not live to enjoy the rewards of her ordeal.

Dr. Christopher's drawing salve, called *German Kermesberro* or *Black Ointment*, has poke root as the primary herbal ingredient and mutton tallow for the drawing effect. With regard to the rather well-known *black and yellow salves*, it is the yellow salve that is the drawing salve. Most such salves also contain beeswax and/or olive oil and some sort of pine tar, pitch, or turpentine. Many formulae for drawing salves can be found in older herb books. Virtually any tallow was used, but for those who object to the use of animal products in their medicines, astringent herbs or clay might be tried—though several physicians in the last centuries advised against using astringents until the malignancy is entirely destroyed. There are laboratories that make healing salves with clay, but many practitioners preferred herbal poultices to clay or tallow-based products since these are safe even if some malignancy remains in the treatment site. Moreover, such poultices do not promote premature closing of the area.

The various formulae for drawing salves exhibited considerable understanding of the patient and his or her process. To limit pain, many of them contained analgesic or anodyne ingredients such as oil of wintergreen or jimson seeds. Some had antiseptic or detoxifying herbs such as barberry or goldenseal. Based on small and preliminary trials, I would suggest that anyone developing such a salve add turmeric to reduce the amount of scarring left by the escharotic process.

HEALING SALVES

Healing salves are used to heal and fill up the holes left when the slough detaches. Drawing and healing salves are both oily; but healing salves do not usually contain tallow, and they do not have the tugging effect of drawing salves. Since they often contain herbs that promote growth of new tissue, such as comfrey root, slippery elm, and mullein, they should probably not be used while malignancy remains in the treatment area. These salves are usually viscous, soothing, and antiseptic. Dr. Eli Jones had a yellow healing salve that he maintained was quite without equal. Hoxsey used a yellow sulfuric powder, a compound he also used on suppurating lesions.

Pattison and Christopher often blended their escharotics with drawing or healing salves. Pattison used a goldenseal paste and calendula ointment in what seemed to be intuitive proportions, depending on the penetration, pain, and separation. Christopher sometimes layered his cayenne escharotic with the black drawing ointment. Hildegard had one formula capable of performing all the actions needed at the various stages of treatment. Her violet salve was rubbed into the area until the entire area was healed.

Not enough is known about the properties of all the herbal ingredients in the various salves nor of the needs of any individual patient. However, *if healing salves are utilized prematurely, the treatment site will close, prevent drainage, and possibly seal residual malignancy in the site*. It should be realized that, due to the use of the escharotic, the treatment area has been traumatized. Dr. John Pattison maintained that this irritation, though necessary, may stimulate the activity, diathesis, of whatever malignancy remains in the area, thereby posing a potentially life-threatening risk.

When a growth appears after surgery, it is termed a recurrence—when it might, in actuality, be the enlargement of what was missed by the surgeons. These same dangers and concerns attend escharotic—and any other—cancer treatment: no part of the tumor should be permitted to remain in the treatment area. Moreover, though I have no medical corroboration of my theory, I suspect that when the hole is permitted to close before all infection and malignancy have been removed, there will be greater scarring and therefore more difficulty with penetration should escharotic preparations be applied again at a later date.

Enucleating Pastes

As we saw in the previous chapter, Dr. John Pattison called his preparation an *enucleating* paste. Enucleation is the removal of a mass from its supporting tissue. This is a fascinating term for many of the salves, but escharotic pastes are not necessarily enucleating since many are not capable of the discrimination necessary to separate malignant from healthy tissue with any degree of precision. Many preparations simply burn—and their producers often do not understand the difference between a caustic and a product that specifically targets malignant cells.

It is worth belaboring this point a bit since lay practitioners often make exaggerated claims for their products. Most of these preparations will lead to the formation of an eschar, and the eschar will detach. However, it is not clear that the entire mass that detaches was malignant—or that all the malignancy is addressed when following the directions that come with such products. To be absolutely fair, when used properly, many of these products can destroy cancer; but they are also capable of making "a mess" of the treatment site without actually finishing the job for which they were provided.

Few patients with whom I spoke described responses similar either to those recounted in historic sources or those claimed by the producers and purveyors of the salves. This may be explained by the fact that the instructions accompanying such products are too sketchy to enable correct use by patients—and more importantly—that the products are not genuinely enucleating. Therefore, more persistence and more aggressive use will simply result in more tissue destruction. The typical escharotic on the market today is a blunt product that can probably remove cancerous masses from the body, but healthy tissue will also be sacrificed in the process. Moreover, these products are considerably more painful than the more selective, enucleating ones.

This said, a few people did report that they discharged masses through the hole created by the escharotic or that pieces detached and fell off onto the bandage. However, when used as I have seen such pastes used, the tumors more often seemed to soften, partially liquefy, and ooze as well as break into pieces that did, of course, separate, detach, and fall out, sometimes over a considerable period of time, from one to seven months.

To be truly enucleating, a salve must discriminate between healthy and diseased tissue and produce a separation of the malignant mass from the healthy tissue. These salves are typically less aggressive than escharotics so a sub-

stance, such as nitric acid, is needed to break through the surface tissue before the enucleating salve can make contact with the malignancy. A salve is potentially better able to make this contact because of its superior penetration as compared to water-based pastes. My understanding is that enucleation is much gentler and potentially quite precise; however, because it is slower than more caustic methods, it is not suitable for fast growing tumors.

As noted, Pattison used an enucleating preparation. He combined goldenseal paste containing zinc chloride with a calendula ointment and said that only one percent of those he treated required additional treatment after the first eschar detached. This is seldom the case with escharotic pastes. Another point in favor of enucleating salves is that they are "quieter." Goldenseal is much less inflammatory than bloodroot. It may even arrest the chemical processes that tumors depend on for survival. Goldenseal is also less painful than bloodroot. Cancer cells have no pain receptors so a treatment that impacts only malignant cells and leaves healthy tissue alone is less traumatizing and probably also safer in the long run. Moreover, any treatment that is easier for the patient to bear will result in higher compliance with the challenges of method.

Because Pattison's formulae and technique are comparatively elegant and gentle, a rather thorough description of his method is provided in chapter 7.

After reading of so many strategies, I am convinced that Pattison and Christopher had procedures that were sensitive and responsive to the patient's need for real healing rather than heroics. If we knew more, it would probably come to light that Hildegard's violet salve was also enucleating rather than escharotic. Interestingly, all three of these practitioners had a profound faith and divine sense of mission that transcended pure medicine.

According to absolutely all of the manufacturers of salves that I have interviewed, the salve will designate an exit unless the patient does so by creating an opening with an external application of an escharotic. If the salve is applied externally, the application site becomes the orifice through which the tumor(s) will exit, this regardless of the actual site of the tumor or quantity of them. This orifice might then be called the *designated safety-valve*. I was told of a woman in Oregon who routinely applies a salve to a spot on her leg to draw out any infections or malignancies in her body. As Johanna Brandt suggested, many people derive a certain comfort from assigning an area to act as a valve through which toxins and other morbid debris can be discharged from their bodies. For those familiar with the salves who have a history of cancer or a fear of cancer, efforts to cleanse the body using the safety-valve approach are often repeated at six- to twelve-month intervals. If nothing morbid exists, it is maintained that there will be no reaction. It is difficult to vouch for the reliability of these claims, but I have used several such products on myself with no reactions whatsoever, this despite the zinc chloride

in the products. This strategy is related more for the sake of completeness than because it is fail-safe.

An anecdotal account may illustrate the usage. A woman who heard about me through a reference in another author's book on cancer telephoned to describe her experience with one of the variations of Compound X (several salves have this name but they are not identical.) Because this story is consistent with others I have heard, I will tell it even if it is a stretch for the imagination for those who are new to the uses of these salves.

> Just before her mother died of cancer, she came to hear of Compound X. She ordered some, but too late to help her mother. The young woman had been roping horses and suffered a severe rope burn when the rope became twisted around her wrists. The burn developed into calluses. At age 23, she decided to try the salve both internally and externally. She experienced some nausea. A variety of masses, the size of peas to silver dollars, discharged through a hole on the wrist created by the salve. She lost some function in the wrist during the discharge process but regained total normalcy some time after the process stopped.

This is a variation of the *safety-valve* strategy. Another variation of the safety-valve method was related to me by the producer of a different Compound X—one whose formula, if my information is correct, is substantially different.

A woman with a lung tumor took an escharotic in tablet form. The tumor chose to exit through the back; as it did so, it forced the ribs to spread. This was quite painful, but a mass the size of a ping-pong ball forced its way, bloodlessly, through the exit it created.

Remembering how I felt when I first began hearing these stories, I can imagine what you, the reader, might be thinking now; but if I had not heard similar reports so consistently, I would have written off these accounts as science fiction. However, documentation of masses having been drawn out through the lungs and skull exist and is proof enough for me at this time.

Variations and Supportive Measures

At the turn of this century, Eli G. Jones, M.D., was probably the foremost expert in the U.S. in the use of escharotics for local treatment of cancer. In his book,[i] he summarized dozens and dozens of case histories along with the local and systemic treatments used. He combined the use of pastes with various poultices and cerates. Regarding the internal treatments as more important than the external, he also used homeopathic and herbal remedies, emphasizing that it is necessary to address the overall constitutional issues, particularly the condition of the blood, as well as the tumor itself.

Unlike those who use salves today, Jones did not use the same protocol for everyone. He determined the type of cancer and developed a strategy for each patient. However, some generalizations are possible. Jones used the gentlest means available given the severity of the growth. In many cases, this meant that a single application of a mild escharotic was possible; in some instances, it meant the use of an aggressive escharotic for six days in a row. The objective seemed to be maximum penetration of the tumor. After he was certain this penetration had occurred, he often followed use of the "black salve" with a poultice made of fresh green poke root and sometimes other ingredients such as crushed lobelia or baptisia (wild indigo) seeds, slippery elm, flax seeds, and bayberry bark. The poultice was (1) changed every two or three hours, or (2) moistened every few hours with herbal extracts or tinctures and changed daily. Jones sometimes used Epsom salts on a white cloth compress; not infrequently, he used cerates (oily substances) with goldenseal, thuja, and poke root. He continued use of such poultices until the tumor detached and fell out. Contrary to the instructions provided by certain lay practitioners today, Jones never used a healing salve until all the malignant material had been removed.

Extraordinary Cases

Just as he was going to press with his book, Jones successfully removed a breast tumor that extended from the clavicle towards the waist, an area seven by eight inches and

---

[i] *Cancer: It's Causes, Symptoms, and Treatment*, 1911. Chapter 8 is devoted to the treatments used by Jones.

two and a half inches at the deepest part. Using half a pound of his No. 4 Paste[j] for each application, he continued this process for a week, changing the plaster daily. He then poulticed the tumor every two hours. The bulk of the mass fell off on the poultice cloth after a week of poulticing.

Since some remaining malignancy was suspected, Jones reapplied his No. 4 Paste for two days, used the poultice for four more days, and another large piece came off. Still not satisfied, he once again applied the No. 4 Paste for another twenty-four hours, used the poultice powder for another week, and was finally satisfied that the entire mass had detached properly. Only when thus certain, he applied *cerate phytolacca* (poke root) three times a day. He described this as a good ointment for cleansing the opening and dissolving any diseased growths that remained in the breast. The enormous wound healed painlessly. At the time of writing, he did not know the prognosis for the patient, but he was optimistic that she would do well because she had also responded nicely to the internal treatments. This was one of the most challenging cases of cancer treated by Jones in his forty years of specialization. It was the crown of a long and successful career.[36]

Several decades later, an equally spectacular use of escharotics was publicly demonstrated by Hoxsey before a full barrage of press microphones and cameras. Hoxsey removed an enormous tumor from the top of the skull of a man who went on to live at least another twenty years.[37]

---

[j] The formula for this is in appendix B, page 192.

MOH'S FIXATIVE PASTE

Frederic Mohs, M.D., is the most recent medical professional to employ escharotic treatments on a large scale. His method is now standard for basal cell carcinomas—for which it boasts a 99 percent success rate. Mohs used the same paste on a wide variety of other types of cancer as well. He called his compound a fixative paste, but it is apparently nearly identical to Hoxsey's escharotic paste.

Mohs described his method in considerable detail and said that chemosurgery permits the surgical removal of the tumor without anesthesia because the fixative paste has killed the tumor by the time surgery commences. According to his book, necrotization of the tumor takes minutes or hours depending on the type of tissue at the application site, the size and depth of the tumor, and the thickness of the application of the salve. After removing a layer of the eschar, he applies more paste and then examines the tissue that has been removed. If he does not "get it all," as determined by microscopic examination, the patient returns the next day for another operation. This process may be repeated for two weeks as he removes tissue, layer by layer. He also uses the paste to arrest bleeding and, as mentioned previously, to define the borders between healthy and malignant tissue. Malignant tissue is more absorbent of the paste; and, after the paste has penetrated the tumor, the neoplasm has a distinctly different color than the healthy tissue, making microsurgery, after acquiring familiarity with the technique, "a nearly intuitive art." After the last surgery, a layer of paste is applied to the open wound which is then bandaged and allowed to heal. There is some scarring, but very little compared to most surgical removals of tumors.

The Mohs method is not a fringe procedure; it constitutes a serious contemporary application and variation of a technique successfully used for countless centuries. It has been studied and reported in reputable medical journals. The book by Mohs contains careful instructions for making the paste, an enormous number of pictures, and diagrams for setting up one's own clinic for performing this work.[38]

SUMMARY

FIRST SALVE	ACTION
Escharotic	blistering
Enucleating	separating
Death by contact	destroying

SECOND SALVE	ACTION
Drawing	pulls out the tumor
Healing	closes the wound

CHAPTER 3

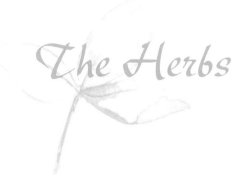

The Herbs

$\mathcal{T}$HOUGH BLOODROOT, *Sanguinaria canadensis*, is by far the most commonly used herb in escharotic salves, many other herbs have also been used with apparent success. Among them are violets, red onions, gold-enseal, poke root, red clover blossoms, blue flag, galangal, lobelia seeds, red sandalwood, cayenne, wood sorrel, and white oak bark. I am certain that this list is in no way complete. For example, I suspect that *fluellin* (speedwell) was used by Nicholas Culpeper in seventeenth century England as well as by the American colonists and that *chelidonium* (greater celandine) was used on the European conti-nent. Recently, I heard of mistletoe being used in an ancient Druid preparation and frankin-cense being added to a black salve made in Utah.

Traditionally, most of the escharotic pastes were made with the fresh roots of the plants or from a concentrate. Today many manufacturers use extracts or powders of roots. A few of the formulae, such as the red clover and wood sor-rel preparations, are made from blossoms that become tar-like after cooking or after being left in water in the sun. With violets, it is also the flowers that are used in the salves though European herbalists report anticancer activity in the leaves as well. Cayenne salves use the pepper, and the Native American roasted red onion formula calls for use of the entire onion along with *puccoon*, which could be goldenseal, yellow puccoon, or bloodroot, red puccoon.

TUMOR DESTRUCTION

Traditionally, professional doctors tended to use acid, such as nitric acid, or mineral caustics containing arsenic[k] or mercury to destroy tumors. Acids are indiscriminately destructive to healthy and malignant tissue alike; they are very painful; and they usually result in the formation of scar tissue. Minerals

---

[k] *The New England Journal of Medicine* reported in its November 5, 1998, issue that arsenic trioxide has been found to be an effective treatment for acute promyelocytic leukemia.

are dangerous because they are absorbed into the blood stream where they circulate throughout the system, resulting in some level of systemic poisoning that is very difficult to correct. As we saw in the first chapter, such a treatment for cancer was mentioned in the Hindu epic *Ramayana*, estimated to have been written 2,500 years ago.

Medical herbalists and lay practitioners, along with a number of physicians and surgeons, have preferred caustics made from plants, usually herbal alkaloids. A few of them combined botanical and chemical medicines by using nitric acid to break through to a deeper tumor; or by adding zinc chloride, a caustic once widely used in cancer treatment as well as dentistry, to a botanical paste; or by adding a toxic mineral to an herbal paste. Since Fell, most of the herbal escharotics have contained zinc chloride; Hoxsey and Mohs both had antimony as well as zinc chloride in their bloodroot pastes.

It should be noted that most authorities, historic and modern, doubt that tumor destruction or removal affects constitutional predisposition to cancer, diathesis. Methods that address only the primary tumor were thus regarded as local as opposed to systemic.

Emetic if taken Internally

What the more popular escharotic herbal salves have in common is that they contain powerful herbal alkaloids that cause vomiting if taken in excessive doses internally. When used externally, small amounts of the herbs and

their active chemical constituents are, naturally, absorbed into the blood stream, but emesis is unlikely due to the relatively minor amount entering the blood stream. Likewise, though toxicity is a concern with a few of the herbs, ingestion of excessive quantities would lead to severe vomiting before a toxic dosage of the herbs could be absorbed into the blood stream. Poisoning would thus be theoretically possible only in the unlikely event that the particular herbs with toxic properties were taken intravenously in substantial excess.[1]

Many of the pastes are provided for internal as well as external use. In small doses, some people have reported—in addition to mild nausea—itching, burning, and tingling sensations at the tumor sites as a result of the internal consumption of the preparations. At the recommended dosage, there should be no complaints of toxicity; however, as a matter of caution, it would be my preference to avoid taking anything internally that contains zinc chloride, this despite whatever claims are made by producers for safety. Zinc chloride[m] is a potent chemical that is not recommended for internal use. One chemist described it as similar to "drinking a drain cleanser."

---

[1] Studies on mice indicate that the amount of poke root necessary to cause death would be quite enormous, much more than is contained in several standard size jars of salve or bottles of the extract. More importantly, few escharotics actually contain poke root though some historic formulae call for the use of poke plasters or compresses, especially for breast lumps. Most of the herbs traditionally used in cancer treatment are not toxic unless taken in very high amounts. Some of the more toxic herbs formerly used in some cancer treatments are now rarely used, and they are not given much mention in this book. These include hemlock, Madagascar periwinkle (used in certain chemotherapeutic drugs), and may apple.

[m] Zinc chloride is made by pouring hydrochloric acid over zinc. It has a pH of 1.8.

For many, internal use is preferred to external use, as it is believed that metastatic lesions are ferreted out and destroyed by the scavenging action of the pastes. To check out these claims, I interviewed numerous individuals who prefer this method of use, either as a stand-alone treatment or as a complement to external applications of escharotics. Many claimed to owe their lives to such use. Though complications as a result of ingestion of the salve are denied by the producers (as well as patients), there is negligible follow-up by most of the people who make and sell the salve.

One medical doctor told of a patient who developed severe gastrointestinal bleeding, although she was uncertain what caused the hemorrhaging as he had combined several protocols without consulting a doctor as to the wisdom of this action. Nevertheless, a few reports of internal uses were astounding: tumors detached and forced their way through the skin despite the absence of any external use (see pages 35-6.)

I decided to test out the claims on myself. I took one of the escharotics that is available as a tablet as well as paste. A few hours after taking a single tablet, I became quite queasy, almost to a point of inability to focus on anything other than the queer sensations in my stomach. This lasted for two to four hours, after which I was quite fine—in fact, substantially more alert and energetic than before. I kept this up for more than a month, one tablet a day, but abdominal distress and reeling sensations attended each use. I discontinued taking the preparation because of my own concerns

for the safety of the method. I did contact the producer. He maintained that, unbeknownst to me, I must be suffering from toxicity. I remain unconvinced. However, like many others, I feel that the herbs are beneficial for a wide range of conditions from congestion to malignancy— zinc chloride is, however, another matter.

TRADITIONAL BOTANICAL ESCHAROTICS

Hildegard said that her violet salve killed cancerous cells on contact. As with bloodroot and poke root, violets can be a powerful emetic; but Nicholas Culpeper wrote in 1649 that they are in "no way hurtful," that they are used to cool heat or are applied as poultices to give relief and dissolve swellings. Modern European sources state that violets are used both internally and externally in the treatment of malignancies and that the leaves, which are also antiseptic, reduce the pain experienced by cancer patients.

Dr. Christopher used the cayenne salve to stimulate circulation. According to most sources, cayenne does not produce anything more than a reddening of the skin when applied to healthy tissue; it is therefore not generally regarded as caustic by herbalists. However, Sam Biser[39] says cayenne ointment stings when it contacts malignant tissues, and Penelope Ody[40] warns that blistering could occur if the ointment is left on too long.

I used Dr. Christopher's cayenne salve on a lump on my ribcage. The pain was "distracting," not unbearable. Within two days, the top of the lump, which was green, separated and fell off. The remainder, which looked like a sebaceous cyst, liquefied and oozed out with a little encouragement from my fingers—which might have been ill-advised had the mass been malignant. I mentioned this to a few friends who tried this salve on similar lumps, even on breast lumps, with similarly successful results. Hildegard's violet salve and Christopher's cayenne salve are genuine salves; and, unlike the water-based pastes, they are rubbed (gently) into the treatment site. If applied frequently, penetration is quite good because of the oiliness.

Since many herbalists seem to think that Christopher's "black ointment" is similar to "the black salve," it important to note that it is not an escharotic but rather one of the more effective drawing salves. His *German Kermesberro Ointment* contains poke root, red clover, chaparral, plantain, and a number of demulcent herbs in a base of tallow, olive oil, and beeswax. Christopher sometimes layered this ointment with the cayenne, but since the salves would tend to blend with each other, even if applied to thin gauze, the method is a bit unclear to me.

Hildegard, who lived in the twelfth century, understood the need to destroy the entire neoplasm and to take tonics to prevent recurrences and metastases. What is disturbing is that centuries later, we seem to be rediscovering information that had been evident to our forebears. It also sometimes seems that medical fashion is not always based on the soundest proofs. It may be modern and endowed with considerable technical explanation, but what happens to mice who have had tumors transplanted into them has never seemed as important to me as what happens to people— with oncogenes predisposing them to cancer— whose growths have arisen spontaneously as a result of factors that, to patients, remain largely mysterious.

FEBRIFUGES

Many of the herbs traditionally used in escharotic salves are classified as *febrifuges* by herbalists. A febrifuge is an herb used to reduce fevers. When such herbal alkaloids are used in inflammatory or perfectly normal situations, they are cooling. I have myself applied two different salves over both small and large areas with no escharotic response whatsoever. In one instance, I had someone apply one of the salves over my entire back; and, as might be expected with a febrifuge, I actually got a small chill, but nothing more.

The initial heat generated when using an herbal escharotic on a malignancy is thus no doubt due to a chemical reaction with the acid at the tumor site since this heat reaction does not occur when the same salve is applied to healthy tissue.[41] Pattison and Snow both discussed the heat reaction. Pattison felt that when one part of the body is warmer than the rest of the body, there will be increased blood circulation to that area: the blood vessels will become distended and with "disease existing there already, the increased supply of blood, must tend rapidly to increase the mischief."[42]

Snow compared the escharotics to regional hyperthermia, indiscriminate burning, noting that we do not know to what extent this action is good and to what extent it is undesirable. In a physician's mind, this kind of localized heat seems similar to, but safer than, irradiation; however, not enough is known to evaluate the risks and benefits of the heat except to note that cancer cells die when subjected to heat.

ACIDITY

The Viennese scientist and two-time Nobel laureate Otto Warburg was celebrated for his work on the impairment of normal cellular respiration (1931). It is now quite well established that cancer cells are anaerobic. There is, according to Warburg, but one prime cause of cancer: the replacement of respiration of oxygen by fermentation of sugar. Absence of sufficient molecular oxygen causes cancer cells to develop into more "primitive" forms that survive on energy produced by the destruction of carbohydrates. This fermentation results in as much as a tenfold increase of lactic acid at the tumor site. Tissue at the site is both acidic and hot, something easily demonstrated by thermography as well as by purely chemical tests. Warburg's primary treatment strategy was to saturate all growing cells with oxygen.

Since most normal metabolic processes of the body tend to produce acids as the end product, there are major theoretical differences between acid caustics and base caustics. It is probable that herbal alkaloids constitute a superior approach to the archaic caustic methods of tumor destruction that rely on acids or toxic minerals. Though purely speculative on my part, it is likely that some of the alkaloidal preparations react with the morbid, acidic tissue in the site of the malignancy and deprive tumors of the energy they need in order to survive. Depending on the particular formulation, the alkaloids may interfere with or arrest fermentation and/or neutralize the acids so that the malignancy becomes inactive and dies. In other cases, the preparations react with the acids in such a way as to produce heat. The heat reaction can be rather minor or quite intense, but it does not last long, some hours to a few days. Since cancer cells are destroyed by heat, death begins to occur when the temperature reaches 104° to 105.8°F. Salve use can, therefore, as Snow suggested, constitute a kind of hyperthermia. The problem is that no one seems to know how warm the escharotic treatment area becomes. However, according to Robert Atkins, M.D., "a relatively small rise in body temperature can make a huge difference."[43] Several pathologists have described the sloughs as "burned tissue, apparently of human origin."

The heat reaction is a somewhat unique characteristic of bloodroot pastes though a few people have described similar experiences with poke root and cayenne. For the record, goldenseal, as preferred by Pattison, is not nearly as inflammatory, even when used with zinc chloride. I suspect that goldenseal has some specific tumor inhibiting properties that rely on its capacity to stimulate immune responses while simultaneously disinfecting the treatment site.

With some preparations, the pharmacology of the herbs may actually be toxic to the tumors in much the same way that chemotherapeutic drugs are purported to be selective in their destruction of malignant cells. Hildegard stated that her violet salve caused death to the "vermes" when they licked it. It is probable that some of the herbs now rarely used in cancer treatment are more toxic to malignant cells than to healthy ones.

Part of the reason for using zinc chloride in the pastes is that zinc chloride penetrates tumors more readily than healthy tissue, carrying with it the other ingredients in the compound. Theoretically, this enhances the specific antitumoral action of the herbs, but no studies of this particular dimension of the treatment are known to me. Mohs reported on the penetration of the tumors, but not on the chemical activity of the individual constituents of his fixative paste and their effects on malignant tissue. Mohs (and Hoxsey) used stibnite, a highly toxic mineral, in addition to bloodroot.

DETOXIFYING PROPERTIES

Warburg's second priority in managing cancer was to protect the cells from further exposure to toxins. Alkaloids are bitter, and according to Ayurvedic medicine, they are cold and detoxifying—and, of course, balancing to acids. Many alkaloids are not just anti-inflammatory or heat reducing, but also anti-infective, antiviral, antibacterial, and antifungal. Goldenseal, the major ingredient in Pattison's enucleating paste, is one of the more highly

respected detoxifying phytopharmaceuticals; and, as we saw in the first chapter, it almost became extinct due to the great demand for it both in the Colonies and in Europe. Its price soared so much that Maude Grieve, a famous herbalist earlier in this century, lamented its increasing lack of availability. Efforts to cultivate it are frustrating, but it is available—even if expensive by herbal standards, over \$200 a pound at our local health foods store.[n]

Another characteristic of alkaloids, according to Ayurveda, is that they have a finer molecular structure than other organic matter. This minuteness enables bitter herbs to penetrate blocked passages and open up channels where other substances are too gross to pass. The opening or decongesting of such channels permits improved circulation so that deprived tissues can receive normal delivery of nutrients and oxygen. Those cells that are not too compromised to recover thus have an opportunity to revert to normal whereas other cells may mature enough to die. This is important because anaerobic cells are immature and do not go through the normal death processes experienced by healthy cells.

Many bitter herbs are liver and blood purifiers, alteratives, and lymphatic decongestants. They are the cornerstones of herbal regimes for improving liver function, reducing infections, and "moving stagnation;" but alkaloids are also neutralizing to acids. This changes the "terrain," an all important condition for pre-

---

[n] Those wishing to cultivate goldenseal can check the author's Web site for an up-to-date list of sources for live roots.

venting proliferation of cancer. Though bitters are essential to good health, Ayurvedic medicine cautions against excessive use of alkaloids because detoxification can be debilitating when carried beyond the optimum point.

However the particular preparations work, reactions are superficially similar. Malignant tissue dies as a result of the chemical reaction and develops into a slough.

When using an escharotic preparation on a malignancy or any other reactive tissue, the process typically begins with a chemical reaction that is variously described as hot, irritating, burning, or blistering. Depending on the formula and method used and the reactivity and sensitivity of the patient, there may or may not be pain. Gradually, the tissue that has reacted with the escharotic necrotizes and begins to form into a slough, discolored tissue that is dead. The size of the tumor, the area covered, and the amount and type of salve used as well as reaction determine how large a slough will form. The slough can be quite small or very large.

When the process is allowed to run its course, the slough will crack around the edge, loosen, and eventually detach from the surrounding tissue in much the way that a scab ripens and falls off. When the treatment is carried out properly, a mass of dead, difficult to distinguish tissue will be cast out from the living tissue. The process is bloodless unless the treatment area has been jarred. Though the initial stages of treatment can be quite painful, the latter stages are more uncomfortable than painful. Most people describe a feeling of weight as the slough feels heavy when it is close to separating from the supporting tissue. This part of the process can take some days to a few weeks depending on the size and depth of the tumor and the product used.

As previously noted, pathologists are not accustomed to examining sloughs. By the time the sloughs are submitted for microscopic analysis, they resist normal descriptions. For the most part, pathologists are only able to determine that the tissue has been necrotized. Only in quite rare instances has anyone been able to detect malignancy. This in no way suggests that the tissue was not malignant— merely that it was burned beyond recognition. A few persons who had biopsies of their tumors before using the salve were unable to obtain confirmation of their malignancies based on the sloughs sent for analysis; but they were, of course, certain that the mass had once been determined to be malignant. In some instances other post-treatment diagnostic tests indicated that the entire malignancy had been removed.

If submitting a slough sample for pathological evaluation, Dr. Snow recommended saving the sloughs in a saline solution such as is used for cleaning contact lenses. When I passed along this suggestion to a friend, her doctor maintained that formaldehyde would have been better. I know people who have tried both methods of preserving the sloughs who still failed to obtain any useful information from their pathologists.

Once the eschar falls off, clean, healthy looking tissue will be exposed. The area could be quite flat or very concave. When a "crater" is revealed, there is usually a small hole at the bottom from which morbid material is discharged, often for weeks or months after the separation of the eschar. It is important at this stage that the site is examined for traces of residual malignancy. If there is even a suspicion of remaining malignancy, the entire process should be repeated. It will generally go faster on the second round.

The hole through which the morbid material is discharged will usually close on its own. It is important not to encourage it to close prematurely because it is releasing debris, some of it quite noxious. Patients tend to feel more and more alert as the body is relieved of this morbid material.

The process may or may not leave scars, although most suppliers of salves will advise their customers that some scarring is likely. The cleaner the site and the freer the individual is of infection, the less likelihood there is of serious, permanent scarring.

FORMULATIONS

The great variety of formulae mirrors the diverse locales and cultural traditions associated with the particular remedies. The use of zinc chloride in combination with herbs was initiated by medical professionals, who, in their search for an effective cancer treatment, combined the best of two worlds: a known caustic with a more harmless, and perhaps more spe-cific, herbal product. Mixing of knowledge for the benefit of those who suffer has no doubt occurred throughout history, and it continues today. Therefore, just as Fell added zinc chloride to the Native American bloodroot treatment, there are today those who have added polymers and dimethylsulfoxide (DMSO) to otherwise perfectly traditional formulae. Whether governed by scientific knowing or a desire to appear more credible or modern to one's patients or peers, the urge to investigate new ideas must have existed as powerfully centuries ago as it does today.

There are products that seem to contain "everything" that has ever been thought to be effective in cancer treatment. For example, an otherwise Great Lakes formula might have chaparral added, but this comes from the Southwest and could not therefore have been traditional for Great Lakes tribes. In some cases, the four main herbs in the Essiac formula have been added to a traditional bloodroot recipe, this without respect to what is generally used internally and what is normally used externally. A few concoctions seem to have come out of textbooks, a bit from here and more from there. They are hence "theoretical" and often completely clinically untested.

Experimentally inclined persons may want to try mixing known anticancer herbs and antimicrobial herbs into proven escharotic pastes. One person discussed green tea extract and tea tree oil in this context, but no trials have been performed on mice or people; it is therefore just an idea. He also suggested trying emu (yes, from the bird) oil because it is an excellent transdermal carrier.

From the vantage point of an amateur anthropologist, I find the modifications intriguing and understandable. If your horse has cancer, why not mention it to the local pharmacist who has probably been dispensing herbs for horses for years? If he mentions three possible strategies, why not combine them all? I did more or less this when my dog had a really nasty and aggressive sarcoma. Kaehi's doctor said that the pain killer was so strong that her gastrointestinal tract would not be able to handle more than a few days of it. After the veterinary prescription expired, I went to Chinatown to get herbal pain relievers. Going from shop to shop, I explained my dog's pain. Besides providing benign but effective pain relievers, the many very helpful and well-informed herbalists recommended all sorts of patent medicines for regenerating bones as well as for treating cancer. I tried everything they suggested, and had any of them worked, I probably would have combined them into one treatment. Perhaps Hoxsey's great-grandfather was luckier, but I suspect the local chemist had something to do with the modifications of otherwise traditional botanical preparations.

Granted, these are just hypotheses, but why would an herbalist use antimony? This is the sort of toxic mineral that traditional herbalists shun. However, a medical doctor, such as Mohs, would have been acquainted with its use and perhaps inclined to experiment until able to develop an effective product. Eclectic physicians were purportedly open to anything that worked, and their publications must have been readily available when Hoxsey and Mohs were young.

Satisfied that the salves have worked for generations, many persons with long-term experience in the use of salves are reluctant to tamper with the formulae. However, those with a grasp of the principles underlying the effectiveness of the salves become artists or even metaphysicians in their use. Pattison was clearly an artist, deeply sensitive to the patient's pain and suffering and perhaps even inspired in the nuances and delicacy of his method. Not only did he blend his enucleating paste with calendula ointment, no doubt to increase penetration as well as reduce spasm, but he used many constitutional remedies that he thought went deeper than the enucleating preparation.

Jones, whose pastes were on the whole quite aggressive and frequently more chemical than botanical, had a number of variations to the basic burn-and-heal strategy. After the escharotics had run their course and the tumor site was open, Jones was persistent in the use of a wide variety of poultices. He used witch hazel, an astringent often contraindicated in the opinion of some of his peers, to clean the site. He also used a camel hair brush to paint liquid extracts of bloodroot or poke root on the tissue exposed after the detachment of the slough. When finally convinced that no more malignancy remained in the treatment site, he used his healing salve to close the area.

Based on what I have come to understand about the use of salves, Pattison and Jones were by far the most accomplished practitioners in the techniques of escharotic treatment.

While their escharotic preparations and techniques differed significantly, they shared professional opinions on other matters: they both held strong views on avoiding surgery; they both used a wide variety of constitutional supplements and homeopathic remedies; they both regarded these as more important than the escharotics; and they both felt that diet plays a role in wellness. In their writings, Pattison came across as a gentle, dedicated healer, Jones as a brave conqueror of a dreaded disease, albeit a knight without a knife!

Though classically trained for his day, Jones parted with authority and developed his own methods of cancer treatment. Jones did not exactly experiment: he was an expert, knew what he was doing and why, and developed remarkable intuition as a result of more than forty years of experience. Like many of his predecessors, he felt that escharotic treatments are difficult and that they belong in the hands of skilled professionals, not inexperienced lay persons.

If professionals were using these methods, I would agree with him; but for the last several decades, this treatment has gone deeper and deeper underground where, as one physician said, "it becomes harder to unearth." Consequently, persons with little or no medical training have become the primary caretakers of the "underground method." Since I have interviewed a large number of these persons, I have to say that I regard all of them as sincere and as genuinely convinced of the efficacy, safety, and simplicity of the products and methods they espouse. However, the other side of this is that after many years of following clues, I do not

have a collection of well-documented case histories that support their beliefs and claims—and all with whom I spoke did, in fact, make claims. This said, I am not suggesting that the products do not work, merely that many who use them are so antipathetic to modern medicine that corroborating material in the form of pathology reports was not sought.

With an occasional exception, I feel that most of the lay products are remarkably similar. However, even after being informed that countless variations of the formulae exist in historic sources, few producers were willing to divulge the ingredients of their preparations, sometimes not even whether or not zinc chloride was a constituent. Almost no one was willing to provide a set of instructions for making the salves; and while I fully appreciate that secrecy has sometimes been necessary to protect the method from extinction, I feel that, given the inability to predict possible allergic and chemical reactions, consumers have a right to more information than the producers have been willing to provide. Moreover, it is quite obvious that humanity is not well served by this kind of withholding of potentially beneficial knowledge.

In general, the purveyors of salves are significantly less trained than their professional counterparts; and most were unwilling to acknowledge the need for greater documentation as to the efficacy of their products. The absence of real proof of the claims for cure made by the producers was, for me, a source of deep discomfort, bordering on the irresponsible.

I found myself faced with a dilemma. I am a strong advocate of more freedom of choice in medicine, and I feel patients have a right to what may work—the more so if their chances are poor with conventional medicine. I am unwavering in this belief. I feel I have a right to participate in the medical decisions that impact me, even in those decisions currently made by others in the name of public safety, but often attended by darker financial motivations. I know there is a movement in some circles towards complete deregulation of medicine. In a "buyer beware" market, there would be little protection for consumers, but there would be a greater flow of information, much of which is legally impeded at this time. Throughout history, such control of thought and knowledge has always been fraught with unacceptable ramifications for the masses. Thus, regardless of motivation, it seems to me best to allow information to circulate as freely as it will. Perhaps the Internet is our current assurance of this. There are, in fact, a number of Web sites discussing escharotic treatment of cancer.

In the meantime, the situation surrounding escharotics is that lay persons are the main sources both of information and supply—and patients are trying to treat themselves and save their lives using products they barely understand and in which they must perforce have the equivalent of blind faith. In most cases, patients using the salves have never met another person who used the same approach; they do not know how to apply the salves or bandage the treatment sites; and they do not know how the salves work or what to expect. They, thus, make a lot of mistakes, partly because they have been given inadequate instructions and partly because, like anything else, skill is acquired through practice in using the methods involved in the treatment. In my view, the time to experiment and acquire experience is best developed before the crisis of illness, but this is not always possible. The present situation is, therefore, far from ideal for the patient; but hopefully this book will encourage more health care practitioners to develop the kind of expertise possessed by Pattison and Jones.

In the meantime, it is easy to understand that hearsay and anecdotal stories by those who keep few, if any, records are not acceptable as scientific evidence. However, in light of the limited success with conventional protocols, even badly documented claims warrant investigation by those with the tools and means to study the methods more scientifically. This is necessary because even, if the clinical success of J. Weldon Fell no longer seems relevant, the Mohs fixative paste and method can hardly be ignored.

As a result of my intrigue with the escharotics, I have quite a list of ideas that, to the best of my knowledge, no one has ever tested. The problem is: cancer is potentially dangerous, so what is known to work in a significant number of cases ought to be tried before experiments with new formulae are contemplated. Nevertheless, Nature offers us an abundance of herbal choices. Hartwell researched 2,500,000 herbs for his book *Plants Used Against Cancer*. An astounding number of them possessed anticancer or antitumoral properties. Thus, if it is known that goldenseal worked for Pattison and bloodroot for many others, we might, using the methodologies of modern herbalism, investigate other herbs, such as *Chelidonium majus* (greater celandine) or coptis, that have similar chemical constituents to see if more common herbs such as these could be substituted for the much rarer and endangered plants used in both historic and contemporary escharotics. However, if attempting such a modification of a traditional formula, it would be wise to try it on a relatively easy to treat basal cell carcinoma rather than on a deep breast lump. If the new formula works, it can be used on other similar malignancies for some years before attempting more heroic uses on deeper tumors; if it does not work, the more proven preparations can be immediately employed to avert unnecessary trauma to the unwanted growth.

There are many possibilities that have not been tried by herbalists, largely because so many of these specialists are discouraged from working with cancer patients due to the virtual monopoly enjoyed by allopathic medicine in this area of medical practice. Nonetheless, given what we know today—as compared to our predecessors' understanding— about cellular metabolic processes and their responses to botanical medicines, there would seem to be ample scope for applying some of this knowledge for the benefit of patients.

PART TWO

Considerations

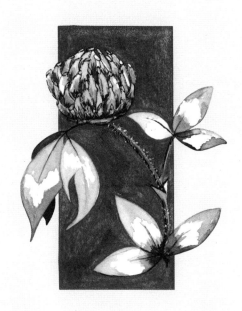

RED CLOVER
Trifolium pratense

CHAPTER 4

Pros and Cons of Salve Use

As noted in the preface, I first heard about cancer salves in 1990. At that time I had already worked in various aspects of healing for two decades, beginning with the mystical and moving towards the physical. During those years I came to know many people who had or had had cancer; and, sadly, I became acquainted with bereaved family members and friends who had lost someone they loved to the dreaded disease. In 1993, I myself lost the person most dear to me to cancer, and soon thereafter, my wonderful white Akita died of cancer. Feeling powerless against disease, I brooded on fate and came to write a book on that subject which is soon to be published.

In my situation as a counselor with a totally holistic view of health and healing, I rarely meet anyone immediately after he or she is diagnosed as having cancer. My work usually begins after all else has failed. I then find myself listening to all too familiar and tragic chronicles of the effort to be cured. Typically, I work with patients who have already had sev-

eral operations, many rounds of chemotherapy, and often radiation as well. In addition, they have sometimes tried a variety of holistic healing strategies including diet, acupuncture and Chinese herbs, various energy balancing therapies, guided visualization, meditation, and frequently some rather complex alternative medical treatments such as are offered in foreign clinics and are not available in the United States.

My sessions with clients therefore usually begin with accounts of the odyssey that has brought them to my door. Unfortunately, I do not offer miracles, merely a wide range of perspectives on constitutional types and temperament and the unique needs of each individual. I help people to understand their own particular stress and emotions and the relationship between their unconscious and conscious selves.

Of the various approaches to the medical dilemma that I employ, there has never been any doubt but that music therapy, whether using live harp music or recordings of classical music, is the most powerful. Though each session is different, insights into personal history and patterns are nearly always forthcoming. In addition, people tend to come into conscious relationship with their souls, their reasons for incarnating, and the gifts that they bring to life. In a few instances, spontaneous remissions have occurred; but these, of course, can never be promised. If such does happen, it is clearly because the time to leave this world has not arrived. In any event, the difficult questions of personal fate tend to be answered in these rather extraordinary, slightly altered states of consciousness.

I am curious by nature. I read and reflect, listen, and ask questions—not only of my clients but of life itself. Where cancer is concerned, I have learned at least as much from patients as they have from me. I am acutely aware that standard cancer treatments are horrific. Not only are they physically maiming but they are also often emotionally battering. In my situation, I tend to meet those for whom these treatments have not worked. I see individuals who have made great sacrifices in the name of cure, who are no longer physically intact, and whose will to live is not matched by therapies that provide better assurance of survival.

Many patients have told me about their experiences in various clinics. Although they may have appreciated the efforts of the holistic practitioners, many were still not free of cancer even after trying a number of alternative treatments. I have spent years studying the various alternatives (1) from the angle of the developer, with whatever biases he might have; (2) with respect to whatever principles underlie the particular methods advocated; and (3) from the perspective of the patient and his or her experience with the treatment. Although I think that many of the complementary methods are indeed reasonable alternatives to surgery, chemotherapy, and radiation, I believe that most single modality approaches are inherently limited. Life involves the entire individual, so healing ought to address the total life experience—not merely the pathology of the particular organism that appears to be threatening life.

As such, escharotic salves are as limited as any of the other therapies. It is therefore important to put their use into a proper perspective. Just as some advocates regard specific diets and dietary changes as adequate responses to cancer, many throughout history have considered the salves as total treatments, and many have urged against such a view. I obviously belong to the latter category. I see that the salves have their place, and probably a far greater place than is currently the situation; however, they are not a cure for cancer. At best, they are an alternative to surgery and perhaps also to chemotherapy and even radiation. Mohs entitled his book *Chemosurgery*, inferring thereby that the paste is both a pharmacological agent and a surgeon. In my opinion, even if some of the salve is absorbed into the blood stream, escharotics ought probably to be considered as local rather than systemic treatments. Cancer salves and pastes are thus better compared to surgery than to chemical treatments.

Though many may not fully agree with me, I think it is reasonable to say that salve use has objectives similar to surgery. In surgery, an attempt is made to remove the tumor with minimal insult to surrounding tissue and physiological function. In reality, this is not how surgery is most often performed since surgeons generally prefer to err on the "safe" side by removing quite a bit more than the tumor itself.

There is perhaps no better example of this kind of "playing it safe" approach than with breast cancer. When I first became interested in cancer, I thought of modern surgery as very technically advanced. I was thus stupefied—no, shocked—to read that the surgical procedure for mastectomies is essentially the same as it was in 1895! As my explorations continued, I learned that many studies have compared mastectomies to lumpectomies and determined that the removal of the entire breast is not necessarily more effective. However, despite a tremendous amount of evidence to support more limited surgical protocols, radical or modified radical mastectomies are still commonly recommended—the argument being that they appear to offer the most scope for addressing metastases to the lymph nodes.

Mohs, famous mainly for his work with skin cancers, actually reported that his microsurgery technique using the fixative paste is highly advantageous in dealing with postoperative recurrences because "mammary carcinomas are invasive and they often extend surprisingly far into the surrounding tissues."[44]

He makes particular reference to the thinness of the chest wall and notes that chemosurgery is indicated because it is "impossible to remove wide margins of normal tissue in this part of the body." The purpose of postoperative use of the fixative paste is clear: if the surgeons miss some of the cancer, the fixative paste is used to destroy what was missed. This is positive indication that Mohs viewed the paste as a sort of chemical surgeon that was capable of tumor destruction where use of the scalpel was impossible or contraindicated.

Contrary to many of his predecessors—such as Fell, Pattison, Jones, and Evers—as well as practitioners using the salve today, Mohs did not recommend chemosurgery for primary carcinomas of the breast. Oddly, his own figures do not support his view. He had limited experience with breast cancer. Whereas he treated thousands of people with cancer, he only saw twenty-two patients with breast cancer; of these, eighteen had suffered recurrences after having had mastectomies. Their recurrences were treated microsurgically using the fixative paste.

While only one of the eighteen women who had postoperative recurrences lived to pass the magical five-year mark, those who were treated for primary carcinomas of the breast using his method fared better. He describes each of the four cases in considerable detail. One patient refused surgery because of fear of pneumonia. Six years after chemosurgery, axillary and distal metastases were found; she lived another year after discovery of these conditions. No follow-up was done on the second patient in this group because Mohs believed her condition to be incurable. With the third patient, "the fungating mass was firmly attached to the chest wall," and the carcinoma was chemosurgically removed. The patient improved enough to enable surgery to be performed, and she lived for six years without recurrence at the primary site. In the fourth case, since it was first believed that the patient had a skin tumor, it was treated chemosurgically; however, it was subsequently found to be a carcinoma. There was no recurrence after three years.

Mohs concludes this section of his book with cautious comments about there not being enough basis for firm conclusions, but that chemosurgery may be effective in removing small recurrent nodules on the chest wall. While his statistics were based on a very small number of cases, it seems evident that those who had chemosurgery were no worse, and seemingly quite a bit better off, than those who had mastectomies.

For some years, except for certain very aggressive malignancies, the standard for measuring survival has been five years. Fell, the American surgeon whose work was reviewed by his London peers, reported mainly on treatments of breast cancer. We do not know the five-year survival rate of Fell's patients. Fell only reported on comparisons between surgery and escharotics after two years. In this time frame, 80% of surgical patients suffered recurrences whereas only 30% of those treated with his bloodroot paste had recurrences of the primary malignancy. These figures impressed

his peers. Jones kept professional records of office visits but seemed to rely on patients to keep in touch with him. Therefore, his long-term survival rate is not certain; we know simply that he successfully removed tumors. Mohs worked in a university where follow-up is the order of the day. Understaffed holistic practitioners do not have the graduate students and grants to perform such research and are consequently short on data. The bottom line, however, is that the salves have repeatedly been deemed effective in breast cancer treatment.

Limitations

In the Mohs technique, there is constant removal of tissue that is readily accessible. His method does not really lend itself to deeper, internal growths. However, some of the more traditional uses of the salve placed no such limitations on its use. Both Fell and Pattison combined an ever so minor amount of "surgery" with their use of escharotics. Fell made little incisions in the dead eschar in order to enable the paste to penetrate deeper. Pattison made scratches for much the same reason. When the escharotic penetrates the entire tumor, the tumor is destroyed. Then, over the course of several days or weeks, the dead mass separates from the supporting tissue and falls away leaving a clean treatment site.

Neither Jones nor Christopher combined any sort of surgery with the escharotic treatments. They relied on the escharotics to penetrate without any surgical intervention. This method depends on the ability of the paste or

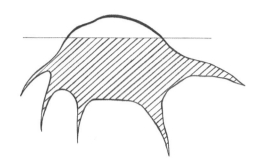

TUMOR MASS PROTRUDING ABOVE THE SURFACE OF SKIN

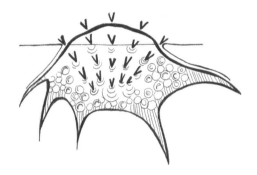

ESCHAROTIC PENETRATING

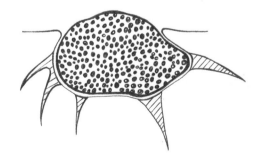

BULK OF THE TUMOR, NOT THE ROOTS, NECROTIZED

salve to necrotize the entire malignancy, to pursue the abnormal cells to the end of the chain described by Dr. Stephen Snow. That the method works is unquestioned, that the escharotics will always succeed cannot be guaranteed. In many cases, treatment is sought too late for anything to be curative.

DIATHESIS

A century before Mohs, surgery was compared to pruning.[45] It was believed that surgical removal of a part of a cancer stimulated the predisposition to further growth. This theory of diathesis, i.e., unusual constitutional predisposition to disease, needs to be understood in the context of surgery as well as escharotic treatment. As it is reasoned in medical science—or rather, as I believe medical science interprets the phenomenon—any exposure of cancer to air tends to make the cancer spread like wildfire. Therefore, once a person is opened up, it is absolutely crucial that the entire malignancy is removed. Whether "pruning" is the problem, or disturbance by the scalpel and air is the problem, is not really known. In any event, Pattison believed that the escharotics traumatize the tumor in such a way that they can cause a reaction that is growth producing, this despite the fact that the tumor had not been exposed to air or cutting. He underscored that the escharotics increase circulation to the treatment site so that the predisposition to growth might be accelerated by the rich flow of blood to the treatment site. This is a risk factor for metastasis as well as growth of the primary tumor.

DIATHESIS
Predisposition to a
particular disease.

Another view—a rather holistic, even esoteric perspective—is that cancer results from metabolic imbalances that favor growth as opposed to catabolic processes. Ayurveda espouses such tenets. According to ancient Indian *pundits* and many others using similar energetic systems of medicine, biological growth tendencies vary from individual to individual—and perhaps also from time to time in the same individual's life. Anthroposophists, following the lead of Rudolf Steiner, believe that the excessive propensity to build is in the placenta at birth. In my own work, I see certain psychosomatic factors that aggravate growth and growth tendencies. For example, grief is anabolic rather than catabolic, more especially so if tears are held within. One might even submit that tumors are the reservoirs of such tears. I am, of course, simplifying; but since detachment of the malignancy may constitute a removal of the reservoir rather than a complete answer to everyone's needs, awareness of such concepts may provide the impetus for some individuals to investigate adjunctive therapies that might enhance their overall health and sense of well-being.

METABOLISM

If the forces of anabolism and catabolism are not in balance, the body suffers the consequences of the imbalance. Constitutionally, anabolic or growth tendencies are either offset by catabolic metabolic processes or they result in surplus: accumulations of fat or deposits. Most practitioners of traditional Eastern systems of medicine—all of which are energetic—do not differentiate between malignant growths and other surfeits such as cysts and swellings. They see all such conditions as metabolic residuals resulting from excess anabolism or deficient catabolism. Modern physicians might recognize weak metabolic functions without acknowledging constitutional types and the various dietary and herbal as well as psychotherapeutic strategies that promote balance.

Since I am usually able to identify such metabolic problems by study of medical and sociological histories, going back to childhood, I basically subscribe to the theory of imbalance as one of the underlying causes of cancer. Long before the cancer is detected, there has been a pattern of imbalance. If this early warning sign had been recognized for what it portended, had the imbalance been properly understood and treated, the diathesis or predisposition to cancer might have remained a tendency rather than an actuality. This theory may be compatible with cutting edge genetic research. A person with certain oncogenes predisposing him or her to cancer should also possess tumor suppressor genes that prevent the potential from becoming a reality. However, a simply enormous array of stressors, environmental as well as emotional, incapacitate the tumor suppressor genes in such a way that the checks and balances fail to work. I hope this discussion encourages some readers to take a wider look at the cancer process.

In the meantime, whereas all may not agree on what constitutes the most thorough and comprehensive treatment of cancer, experts do agree that it is important to remove or destroy the entire neoplasm. What is thus needed is a method that can achieve this goal with maximal safety and minimal distress and loss to the patient. As such, I feel that escharotic treatments deserve consideration. First of all, they do not "cut." There is no severing of nerves, no loss of body parts, no blood loss, and no interference with how the lymphatic system operates to remove debris from the body. Against these trumps, the matter of how best "to get it all" has to be factored into the decision-making process. In terms of the escharotics, the main obstacle to total tumor destruction or enucleation is lack of perseverance. Other drawbacks have been lack of skills and understanding of how and why the salves work, faulty instructions for use, as well as a greater or lesser ability to deal with pain.

Pain

Most of the products presently supplied by salve producers are challenging to use. Pain is a major deterrent to use; however, no two salves and no two patients are alike. Some escharotics are more intense than others, and some people have higher pain thresholds than others. Moreover, where there are more nerves in the treatment site, there will obviously be more nerve sensation; but even for the same patient, reactions are not the same throughout the entire course of treatment.

This said, reactions to the escharotics vary from an increase in circulation and swelling in the application site to itching and burning to intense pain. However, as noted, the fact that one application hurts nearly unbearably does not mean that subsequent applications will be as painful—nor is it true that because the first application is relatively painless that subsequent applications will also be. In short, no predictions are possible.

I have spent eight years brainstorming the pain issue. In some of the historic literature and testimonial statements, there is reference to painless removal of malignancies. Today, no such assurance is provided by the salve producers.

Interestingly, nearly all the primary herbs used in the escharotic pastes have pain relieving properties. Several of the herbs belong to the poppy family and are hence intrinsically sedative. Others have dulling properties.

Pattison prescribed codeine for pain and nepenthe, a form of morphine, for sleep, though he stated that, with his method, most of the nerves are deadened by the time the reaction intensifies. Mohs sometimes used morphine. One medical doctor who uses the salve in her practice says that it is sometimes necessary to anesthetize the area with lidocaine or procaine. One patient who used the salves was married to a pharmacist who gave her prescription pain relievers. Other patients have saved pain pills that were previously prescribed for pain unrelated to salve use.

I believe all these to be reasonable solutions, but I have searched for more natural ways to manage the pain, methods patients can themselves use without the need for prescription medication. Native Americans put jimson seeds in their salves; these are toxic, but so are many things in our world today, and not much is required. Jones used *corydalis*, turkey corn, in both homeopathic and herbal forms for cancer cachexia (the wasting syndrome associated with cancer). Corydalis is a Chinese remedy used to invigorate the blood and relieve pain, but I know patients who tried corydalis without sufficient relief. So far as the homeopathic pain remedies go, I doubt that people today respond as dramatically to homeopathic remedies as they might have at the turn of the century when Jones was in practice, but I leave this discussion to homeopaths.

As an aside, but relevant to the pain problem, I was recently bitten twelve times by a black widow spider and was in excruciating pain for the better part of a year. I tried "everything." Most pain relievers compromise the functioning of the gastrointestinal tract, but there are some herbs—herbs that I discovered while searching for relief for my dog—that do not have this side effect. They had helped Kaehi significantly, and I had some remaining after she died. They worked quite well for me, but they did induce drowsiness.

Unfortunately, the stronger and more effective herbal pain relievers have been appropriated by the pharmaceutical industry and are no longer legal for use in herbal products. This infuriates me, but this is not a book about the economics and politics of medicine. There are, however, some herbs that can legally be added to the salves, without inhibiting the action of the salve, herbs that give long-term pain relief. White willow bark and pseudoginseng are two such herbs. A number of essential oils, such as clove, eucalyptus, wintergreen, and some forms of thyme, reduce pain, at least temporarily. Many of these herbs are found in ointments for muscle soreness; but for the salves, it is necessary to use something with very deep and long action. Some Chinese martial arts preparations, called *di da wan*, have provided up to fourteen hours of pain relief.

To understand this matter, try imagining a treatment using a caustic acid or electric heat device; it would be unbearable and constitute torture. Because the herbs in the salve are actually cooling and sedative, it is most likely the zinc chloride that is the cause of most of the truly severe pain—though, admittedly, it is not an ingredient in all of the escharotic preparations. It was not a constituent in the cayenne salve that I used, but it was in many of the pastes I applied to myself as an experiment. When zinc chloride is part of the escharotic, it may make up anywhere from two to fifty percent of the paste by weight. If the tissue does react, reactions can sometimes be fierce, even if part of the potential pain is masked by the herbal anodynes. I have discussed some possible solutions to the pain issue with a few salve producers in order to help them develop more tolerable products. I have no financial interest in this, but pain is a major deterrent to escharotic use and a major cause of lack of compliance and abortion of the process midstream, something that is not recommended by those familiar with the process. Most salve producers are totally dedicated to their work, so overcoming the pain issue will remove the biggest objection to their products.

On the other side of this consideration of pain, it must be said that most people using the salve report that they are able to function during the day with an aspirin or codeine, but they do not sleep at night. I used one of the salves on an undiagnosed lump on my rib cage. It hurt a lot but was not unbearable. I was teaching a seminar, and no one in the audience seemed to notice anything unusual in my manner though I knew I was in pain. The pain was not incapacitating, not nearly as bad as the spider bites! Others have compared the pain to toothaches, childbirth, fractures, and even surgery. Most said that these more familiar sources of pain are worse than those brought about by escharotic use.

To determine whether the pain of escharotic use is too excessive to warrant use of this method, several factors have to be considered. First, the pain occurs only with the use of the escharotic itself, not with the poultices, cerates, drawing, or healing salves. Since there are many ways to use these products, it is difficult to say how much pain there will be or how long it will last. The worst I have heard is that the pain lasted for two to three days after discontinuing use of the escharotic. Usually, the pain begins to subside as soon as the salve is removed. If the response to the escharotic is slow, no pain is felt in the early stages of use. So, if it takes three days to produce a visible sign of a reaction, there will not be pain until the area starts to blister. Then, since there are various methods of use, the escharotic may only be applied once or it may be applied six or even ten times, either all at once or interrupted by the use of other products.

The amount of pain involved in removing a small skin tumor is so negligible that only the most fearful patients need avoid this treatment. With larger tumors, such as occur in the breast or liver, pain will probably be intense for a total of a week or so, either seven days spread out over two months or seven days in a row. Compared to the pain of surgery or chemotherapy, this is not extreme—nor is it similar to irradiation in that at most there will be some scarring, not residual pain in the treatment site.

SCARRING

The other problem with salve use is that virtually all of the salves leave scars. It will be remembered that one of the definitions of escharotic is "scar forming." How much scarring occurs may depend on a number of factors: acidity of the tissue at the application site, infection, and how rapidly the treatment site is allowed to close. Aggressiveness of the particular escharotic and its ingredients no doubt also affect this matter.

Since the herbal escharotics are alkaloidal, they neutralize the acidity surrounding the malignancy. However, because of the addition of zinc chloride to most of the preparations, the overall pH of the paste may be acidic. One of my sources indicated that the pH of the formula he makes is 3.7–3.8. Zinc chloride has a pH of 1.8 and is 50% by weight in his formula. Many of the products are probably more alkaline since they either do not contain any zinc chloride or they contain much less than the

CERATE
Oily substances for external use, usually made with fat or wax.

one made by this particular person. Pattison used 25% zinc chloride in his enucleating paste, but he only used one part enucleating paste to nine parts calendula ointment on the first day of treatment with the paste. Zinc chloride therefore constituted only 2–3% of the total preparation at that early stage of treatment.

Since most of the alkaloids in the escharotics are also anti-microbial, they will, if used correctly, reduce whatever infection is already present. If the site is completely free of morbidity before the area is permitted to close, scar formation is minimal. For this and other reasons, the suggestions throughout this book can be used in lieu of those provided by the producers of the salves.

Adding turmeric to escharotic as well as to healing salves also greatly lessens scarring. Turmeric is antiseptic, emulsifying, and antitumoral. Its use protects against infection while also reducing scarring. Turmeric can be taken internally and applied topically in ointment form for months following treatment until the scars are all but invisible. There are a number of other scar removal products available. They are discussed on my web site.°

It should be remembered that surgery also leaves scars. Many surgical incisions do not heal properly because the patient is not well enough to heal. Moreover, since recurrences often involve surgical scar tissue, it is crucial that patients and practitioners take a more serious look at scarring than heretofore. I have seen some very worrisome scars, and some of the strategies mentioned in this book may help patients who have not healed to deal with the side effects of infections and operations, even if the problems began many years prior to proper treatment.

PATIENT INVOLVEMENT

In considering the pros and cons of escharotic treatment of cancerous masses, one needs to address the issue of "doing it yourself." Most patients with whom I have spoken have had a lot of questions as they entered different stages of their processes, and they were understandably often frustrated by lack of information concerning the dramatic changes occurring to their bodies.

Lack of qualified support and shortage of answers concerning individual nuances of response to the salve are definite cons. Weighed against these issues are what many describe as a major pro: they have taken charge of their own healing. For them, this is a source of empowerment. Control over what happens to the body is restored to the patient who is not only directly involved in the treatment but also usually mesmerized by an absolutely fascinating process, a process that provides daily evidence of the fact that morbid matter is being discharged from the body. Even physicians are intrigued by the process. One jested with me that she is selling tickets to her colleagues to view the treatment site during dressing changes.

This said, on the other side of the subjective value of being more in charge is the objec-

---

° http://www.cancersalves.com

tive fact that few patients actually know what they are doing when they take charge of their own healing. This can be risky and therefore often foolish and disappointing.

RELIABILITY

Another issue relating to this discussion of pros and cons is not supervision, but assurance. There are two main concerns falling under this topic. The first has to do with the reliability of the method, and the second focuses on follow up procedures that determine whether or not the patient is cancer free. As for the safety and success of the method, much has already been stated. Escharotic treatments appear to be at least as successful as other cancer treatment methods. Moreover, the need for some way of determining whether or not a patient is cancer free is essentially the same regardless of the treatment used.

POST-TREATMENT DIAGNOSTIC TESTS

So far as "evidence" goes, there are patients who do not have a need to know. Once they have seen the masses detach and they no longer feel lumps in the tumor site, they are satisfied that they are out of the woods. Others want follow-up confirmation that the cancer has disappeared. In such instances, there is no doubt much room for argument as to what would constitute the most infallible determination. With some forms of cancer, such as prostate and ovarian cancer, there are reliable blood

tests. I personally prefer dark field microscope examinations or the Antimalignin Antibody in Serum (AMAS) test, a very simple, non-invasive blood test with a high level of accuracy, but few physicians seem to know about either of these tests. In any event, after a mass has been removed, it seems unnecessary to have more mammograms, MRIs, needle biopsies, and such; but this is a matter of individual choice—and clearly a choice upon which life may sometimes depend.

Reasonably speaking, all persons who have had cancer at any time as well as those who may be genetically predisposed to cancer or specially at risk of cancer because of exposure to agent orange or asbestos or radiation or any of the zillions of other carcinogens in our environment are faced with the same diagnostic challenges. How can one detect cancer before it spreads?

At this time, we simply do not have adequate means for determining the existence of cancer. Personally, I believe that we are living in such a dangerous time that all any of us can do is make healthy life style adjustments and adopt sane preventative measures while also committing to routine maintenance such as periodic detoxification regimes to compensate for the pollution and other hazards to health to which we are all exposed.

RECURRENCE AND METASTASIS

Perhaps the most disheartening aspect of cancer is its proclivity to recur. This tendency is well noted and undenied by allopathic and

AMAS

This test can be ordered from Oncolab Inc., 36 The Fenway, Boston, MA 02215. Telephone: 617-536-0850 or 1-800-9CA-TEST. Oncolab Limited in Britain: 93 Harley Street, London W1N 1DE. Telephone: 01-486-0923.

holistic practitioners alike. Though there are many speculations as to why cancer develops in the first place, and somewhat fewer theories as to why it recurs, recurrence is the nightmare of every patient. Patients are seldom told that regardless of whether or not they have surgery, irradiation, or chemotherapy, cancer has a nasty way of reappearing, often in the scar tissue of the surgery incision. Technically speaking, recurrence is the reappearance of the same type of cancer in the original site, the place of the primary tumor.

Metastasis is the other major issue faced by patients. Cancer cells migrate from their place of origin to remote parts of the body via either the lymphatic system or blood stream. A metastatic cancer may exist before the primary cancer is even found—and it may be undetectable at the time the decision is made as to whether or not to operate. In theory, surgery will not be curative if a metastatic cancer has established itself, even though this cancer may be too small to detect at the time the primary cancer is discovered. To wit, only a systemic treatment can possibly succeed if metastases are present, and the only systemic treatment offered by conventional medicine is chemotherapy. Its cure rate is so low that it is practically immeasurable except in the case of a few childhood cancers, leukemia, and some forms of Hodgkin's disease.

Patients are seldom given these facts until conventional treatments have failed. Though surgery is, without doubt, the best weapon modern medicine has against cancer, it is drastic. It does not address either the cause that first gave rise to the malignancy, or the possibility that the cancer has already infiltrated the neighboring tissue or broken away from the primary tumor and metastasized. Radiation is supposed to be able to destroy enough of the tissue surrounding the tumor to obstruct the pathways by which metastasis may occur; however, it also causes ulceration and burns of perfectly healthy tissue and interrupts the systems that supply nutrients to tissue. Moreover, it is quite well accepted that radiation often causes secondary tumors, i.e., malignancies that were not related to the original tumor.

Arguments for or against any option are many. Ultimately, all anyone can do is evaluate the premises of each technique and strategy, measure the risks against the strengths of each, and then decide which risks are acceptable and which side effects are not. This said, it should be realized that wherever there is injury to tissue, the body will exert itself to repair the damaged tissue. If the site that is mutilated contains abnormal cells, the odds are that these, too, will multiply—not only those performing repairs. The holistic approach would thus be to avoid measures that further traumatize the injured area. As such, it may also be important—at some stage of the treatment—to provide the nutrients that are needed to protect and repair the tissue that is damaged.

PRECISION

Most exponents of salve use believe that the salves discriminate between healthy and diseased tissue in such a way as to destroy only the malignant and infected cells. "Self-biopsying" is the term used by some. Video footage in my possession illustrates this point exquisitely. An angiocentric T-cell lymphoma had wrapped itself around a large artery on the face. At one point, the artery was exposed to view; it was remarkable how well the herbal "mop up" had proceeded. The site was, as always with the escharotics, bloodless and cleaner than even the most skilled surgeon could have left it.

Hoxsey claimed that his yellow powder was selective; however, neither trichloroacetic acid, which was presumably used to break through the skin, or his red paste (containing antimony trisulfide, zinc chloride, and bloodroot) were capable of discriminating malignant from healthy tissue. Clearly, it is important to know exactly what is in the external preparations before making assumptions as to how they will work.

INTERNAL TONICS

If the salves really work as accurately as some believe, it would explain the relatively low recurrence rate reported in historic sources. The use of elaborate adjunctive body site-specific protocols, as described by Jones and Christopher, may also help account for the wonderful healings reported by these doctors. Among the many holistic practitioners using escharotic treatments, they alone described the internal herbal remedies they used for each organ system—and they always recommended that these be used whether or not the escharotics constituted part of the treatment.

It is important to realize that there is always a cause behind effects. Tumors are effects. Destruction of a tumor does not touch the cause. If the cause does involve excessive mitotic activity because of irritation, constitutional predisposition, or other factors, then the growth-inhibiting herbal preparations, such as those containing alkaloids, would seem to offer more promise than other therapies in vogue today. For example, turmeric, a culinary spice with no known toxicity, has shown these properties in laboratory tests. In theory, cytotoxic drugs (chemotherapeutic agents) are growth-inhibiting, but so extremely poisonous that at a certain point, the drawbacks to their use outweigh whatever advantages there might be to such drugs. There are nontoxic herbal protocols that may be more effective in the long-run because of the patient's ability to tolerate the dosages better than chemotherapy.

DETOXIFICATION

Once an opening is made by the salves, various purulent matter will ooze from the site. This may be clear, whitish, yellowish or greenish. While it is often assumed that most of these discharges stem from systemic maladies, impaired circulation may account for some of the morbid deterioration of tissue in the cancerous area. It is not clear that everything that comes out is cancerous. It is, however, worth noting that the escharotics are active in fighting infections as well as cancer. Mohs used his paste to treat gangrenous conditions as well as cancer.

It is also important to note that tumors are toxic. If they are left in the body, they either grow or are destroyed. If they die, they have to be disposed of by the eliminatory systems of the body which are then often quite overtaxed, especially if they are killed as a result of cytotoxic drugs. With salve use, not only is the tumor removed, if it is properly enucleated, but a hole is created through which other morbid matter is discharged. When patients undergoing this treatment are observed, it is apparent that—even if preoccupied with and even obsessed by the treatment—they become more alert as the process progresses. Their coloring improves, their vitality increases, and their attitudes usually brighten as well. Discharging toxic material in this way is obviously easier than burdening the lymphatic system, liver, and kidneys with detoxification. This is certainly one major argument in favor of salve use.

PROFESSIONAL ASSISTANCE

A common deterrent to salve use is the concern on the part of some patients that, if they pursue an alternative course of treatment, there will be no one to whom they can turn if "something goes wrong" during the treatment itself. Though escharotic cancer treatment is relatively safe, lack of trained and experienced persons to assist with the process is a definite negative weight on the list of pros and cons. We can only hope that as more people become acquainted with the method that the shortage of expertise will be corrected.

Patients are also often afraid that if they do something their primary care physicians or oncologists do not understand, their doctors may refuse to perform normal diagnostic tests to determine whether the cancer has, in fact, regressed or disappeared, or their doctors will abandon them in case of emergencies. The fear of being left high and dry in case of real medical need discourages some patients from undertaking a treatment that is not prescribed by their physicians.

Personally, I feel that some of these anxieties may be exaggerated, but there is no doubt that some doctors do give rise to the impression that their compassion is reserved for compliant patients. It must be obvious that no one desires an adversarial relationship with someone upon whom he or she may at some point depend for support. Still, there are doctors who themselves are seeking alternatives that offer the patient more hope and spare them distress. In my position, I am, of course, more likely to meet such doctors than their more conservative colleagues. In any event, I acknowledge that, because of their need for support, some patients have made decisions based on what their doctors advise rather than on what they themselves prefer.

It should, of course, also be noted that perfectly well-trained doctors may not understand what they see when viewing an escharotic treatment site. One patient who commenced escharotic treatment on his own went to a foreign clinic where they tried to rub off the eschar. Other patients have been warned of the risk of infection by doctors who are not conversant with the anti-infective properties of the botanical preparations. Still others have been scolded for trying something without proper supervision. The solution for this problem is good relationships with open-minded doctors.

after irrevocable procedures had been performed. Though not entirely convinced that the escharotics are self-biopsying to the extent sometimes claimed, they do not cause either the side effects or irrevocable losses typical of conventional cancer treatments.

DIAGNOSIS

Another subject affecting choice of treatment is the reliability of the diagnosis. Many years ago, someone in our meditation group went to the hospital for what she hoped would be a simple fibroid procedure; but, in the event that something worse were to be found once she was cut open, she placed elaborate constraints on the surgeon. I waited outside the operating room with her partner. Hours went by; we finally got word that there was massive malignancy that had infiltrated "everything." For more than half a year after this, tissue samples were still being sent to one expert after another. It was malignant, it was not; it is, it is not. She never did know which, if any, of the various opinions she could trust; and she was unwilling to base her decisions on judgments over which there was so little accord. She therefore did not agree to more radical surgery. She is still alive.

Certain patients who have experienced cancer treatment have come to fear doctors and hospitals. After being diagnosed with cancer and following the recommended procedures, they either discovered that the treatments had failed to cure them or that what they had was not, in fact, malignant—this

TREATMENT OF THE APPEARANCE

In my study of older herbal and medical books, I found that historically the treatments for ulcerations, exudations, and malignancies were essentially the same. Following in this tradition, many salve producers see their products as panaceas for everything from a simple planter's wart to metastatic cancer. The various discharges from the application site are interpreted as liquefications of tumors or pus, but few seemed inclined to seek verification of their assumptions by a pathologist. If satisfied that these distinctions would not affect treatment decisions, there is perhaps no need for substantiation of diagnoses via normal tests. When I had a lump, I did not feel impelled to have the mass analyzed as I was quite certain that, regardless of its pathology, I would treat the lump in the same manner; however, I fully recognize that others have far more need for facts. They should therefore act in accordance with their particular informational requirements.

Since we are not living in a time of ideal medical diagnoses and protocols, we have to form our judgments based on the information available and make our decisions accordingly. Personally, I have never had a "need to know" what is going on in my own body. If something is amiss, I try one thing; if it doesn't work, I try something else. Other people are more nervous and feel that cure is not possible without first getting the right label for a condition. I do not see treatment or cure as dependent upon a label but rather upon the symptoms. Still, I recognize that even though some physicians hand out antibiotics before getting laboratory results, doctors generally require a diagnosis in order to proceed with treatment. With energetic systems of medicine, treatment is based more upon symptoms than pathological proofs. Therefore, if I have a gland that is swollen, I take herbs to boost my immunity and stimulate lymphatic drainage. I am comfortable with these strategies, but not everyone else is.

Thus, each individual facing major medical issues and the need to make decisions needs ultimately to find a reasonable balance between facts and safety, as measured by outer criteria as well as more subjective standards, such as the willingness to undergo the measures needed to achieve health and to be at peace with one's decisions. This is harmony, but it is elusive in most medical situations today.

Science and Credentials

Absence of proper scientific information has to be weighed against the logic just stated, but science does not have all the explanations either. Even in fully equipped and highly sophisticated medical institutions, questions cannot always be answered; and even with state of the art diagnostic equipment, oversights and mistakes are made. I certainly know people whose lumps were dismissed as harmless when no corroborative evidence was sought and others who have had major procedures that were later found to have been unnecessary. This is not professional, but it happens every day regardless of training, credentials, and licenses.

This said, it is important not to skirt the issue of whether or not escharotic treatments really address cancer, or whether bone spurs, warts, and lipomas are being confused with life-threatening cancer. For me, though some self-diagnoses are probably wholly lacking in factuality, the preponderance of evidence favors the belief that cancers are also destroyed by the pastes when they are used properly.

Moreover, as one patient put it, this was the only treatment that drained toxins from her body. All others had compromised certain functions in the name of cure. What every patient needs is enough information to make an informed decision. What works for one patient may not have the same effect on another. If not trained in medicine, it is sometimes difficult to trust important decisions to oneself. This is why people consult specialists. This book may provide enough material to fill some of the informational gaps and spur others to greater investigation of the many dimensions of this treatment so that, in the future, experts will be more easily located.

CHAPTER 5

Testimonials

As shown in the first chapter, escharotic treatment of cancer has been continuous for the last 2,500 years. Though mineral caustic preparations are truly passé, botanical treatments have earned the lasting respect of patients and practitioners. In the United States, these herbal remedies were at one time as well known as first aid remedies are today. In rural areas of the Carolinas, Tennessee, Oklahoma, and the Rocky Mountains, use of the pastes remains popular and has the distinction of appealing almost equally to both lay and professional practitioners. While lay use of escharotics remains a rather simple albeit often effective approach to cancer treatment, naturopathic doctors as well as physicians and surgeons have, during the last hundred and fifty years, developed extraordinary expertise in the method.

Some people naïvely attribute almost miraculous properties to the pastes, but more cautious professionals have also been convinced that escharotics are the safest and surest way of removing tumors.

When first questioning people about the salves, I was miffed by the secrecy surrounding the products. However, since publication of the earlier editions of this book, more and more people have discussed their experiences with the treatment. In the hopes of sparing humanity from unnecessary suffering and premature death, a few have divulged their recipes. Sadly, fear of unwanted media attention and/or reprisals by officials of the Government has made others unwilling to talk.

I am personally certain that, at minimum, escharotic treatments offer improved quality of life to those suffering from cancer. This is partly because of the relatively less invasive—as compared to surgery and radiation—manner in which they work and partly because of the way they provide an outlet for detoxifying the body. To this extent, botanical escharotics are a genuinely natural treatment, but I am not persuaded that they save lives unless very skillfully used. Yet, when thus used, they constitute an acceptable alternative to conventional treatments.

For me personally, the research for this book has been fascinating and frustrating. Many of my academic interests have been combined into one study: medical history, anthropology, ethnobotany, and cancer cure; and the process has been an adventure as well as a sometimes not so pretty window into history. The most vexing part of trying to report this treatment factually has been the absence of solid evidence. Properly documented cases probably exist, but this treatment has for some reason tended to travel the testimonial route.

I believe this is due to one main factor: official disregard so that the method has been kept alive by lay practitioners rather than professionals. Botanical escharotics are the option they are today because their use has been perpetuated by non-professionals, by sincere individuals who, for the most part, lacked training in medical herbalism and medicine. Hoxsey was the most prominent of these persons, but there have been and continue to be others who never acquired Hoxsey's high profile.

Because the testimonial tradition has been the mainstay of information about escharotic treatments over the last century and a half, it is appropriate to provide a few samples of letters from patients. As will be seen, they illustrate a fairly consistent pattern of patient gratitude.

Patient of T. T. Blake, M.D., New York, 1858[46]

The growth was entirely removed and had healed in three weeks. There was little pain connected with the treatment which also consisted of internal medication to purify the blood.

GIDEON LANGDON

Patient of Dr. Perry Nichols, Savannah, Missouri, 1929

In June, 1924, I became afflicted with cancer in my mouth, involving my left lower gum and spreading to the cheek. Being somewhat versed as to the nature of the disease, as I am an M.D., I knew that something had to be done. Like most other doctors I sought that which I thought was the most reliable treatment, and consulted a firm of doctors in whom I had perfect confidence; men whom I knew to be thoroughly reliable, and whose reputation as specialists is surpassed by none in the Southwest.

They began giving me the radium treatments and apparently were in a fair way to make a complete cure of my trouble. I visited their offices every six to eight weeks for almost three years. The last application of radium was in April, 1927, and after that, I became so much worse than at any time before, that it seemed that I could not live but a few days.

In January, 1927, a party told me of the Dr. Nichols Sanatorium at Savannah, Missouri, and advised me to go there, but like most doctors I was skeptical of anything pertaining to the treatment of cancer by Escharotics. However, when I had finally reached the point where I knew I had to have relief from the suffering and disease, or not live long, I wrote to the Dr. Nichol's people and received a very courteous letter in reply and also one of their books.

By this time, I was unable to lie down, and for eight weeks, sat in a chair day and night. When I got the book I read it carefully and wrote several people whose names I found listed as cured patients and with whom I had a personal acquaintance. Their replies were so uniformly enthusiastic, that I finally started to Savannah, Missouri, in June, arriving there more dead than alive, it seemed to me.

By this time I was suffering such extreme pain that I had Tetanus starting in, and when I presented myself at the office of the institution for examination, they could hardly examine me and gave me but little encouragement as to the final outcome.

My statement was, in reply to their prognosis of 40%, that I knew my time was limited anyway and that I desired them to do what they could. They began the treatment the next morning and in just seven days the cancer was removed, taking away more than half of my left cheek. In three weeks from the day I entered the Sanatorium, I started home with no trace of the cancer remaining.

However, I was home just fourteen days when I discovered a necrosis of the bone caused from radium and returned to the institution. They removed about two inches of the lower jaw bone. From then on I have had no more cancer trouble. Just about a month ago I again entered the institution for plastic surgery to close the opening in my cheek. At this time the wound is healing nicely and I feel that I am well once more.

These people are effecting cures that I did not think could be done and I had ample opportunity to observe what they are doing for I was shown every courtesy by the doctors in charge. I earnestly advise every one who has cancer to consult these people, as they will tell you honestly if, in their opinion, you can be cured or not.

This testimonial is being given by me without any solicitation on the part of any one connected with the Sanatorium, and with the hope that it will induce someone who needs their help to go to these people for treatment.

A. R. HUGHES, M.D.
AMES, OKLAHOMA

CONTEMPORARY LETTERS
FROM PATIENTS

Letter to D. R.

Forgive me for not writing sooner. This has been a very traumatic experience for me. It started when the doctor did biopsies on two spots on my nose. When the results came back from Michigan University Hospital, he told me that I had cancer. The doctor wanted to put me in the hospital that day, but the dread for me was so great that I twice put off going. It got worse during those two weeks of procrastination. I knew I had to make a move. That was the day I met you folks at the coffee shop. After I talked to you, I began to have hope that I could fight cancer another way.

I have been house bound, prayerful, and busy since receiving your salve. I started the treatment on December 2nd. I appreciate being able to call you and our friend in North Carolina. I shall never forget the two of you. I didn't know if I could do it alone; but with your support, it worked.

Here is how it went:

Day 1: The initial application was applied on Monday at noon. I applied the salve to the two spots the doctor had determined to be cancerous. I packed the two spots full of salve.

Day 2: The salve was pulling and drawing but not painful.

Day 3: My face and the cancer sites were swollen.

Day 4: My eye was badly swollen. The skin was red and festering. Pussy looking toxins were oozing out of the area, like a glass of milk was thrown in my face.

Day 6: I was amazed to see the whole left side of my nose eaten away to the tip of my nose, so I packed the nose from the tip to the bridge with salve. I also added fresh salve over the old salve.

Day 7: Still pulling and drawing. White drainage was coming out of the hole in the nose where a large scab began forming. I could see deep inside my nose. When the scab came off, I found only a small hole where the core was.

After that, I went through the process of hydrogen peroxide, Vaseline,^{TM} and bandages. My nose has filled in fairly well. I am hoping for more to come so the scar will be less, and I won't need any (reconstructive) surgery. It is now one month and one week since I started. There is some red mess there pulling so I'll keep on as long as I need to. I'm glad I used the salve.

March 12th: I have only a small scar, and it seems to be disappearing.

Thanks!

Letters to I. N.

Dear Ingrid,

I am so thankful that the salves exist. As a result, I have a husband and a son that I wouldn't have had, had it not been for the salves.

/B.T./

Dear Ingrid,

We received your wonderful letter yesterday and I wanted to respond as soon as possible. I have been thinking about writing you for several weeks—to share with you some of my experiences using the salves. It is my hope that the following could be of use.

My whole experience using the salves could be characterized by the words, AWE, GRATITUDE, and MIRACULOUS. Seeing as how I am still in the midst of the process, everything I say should be qualified with the words "so far." It would be unwise, it seems to me, to jump to any final conclusions, as no one can tell what the future will bring. I am respectful of the Great Mystery operating through all of us. Yet I feel confident telling you about my experience "so far." It has certainly been a great adventure.

Even before I spoke to you, Ingrid, and found out about the salves, something important happened. I had had lumps in my breasts for a long time—they never seemed to get bigger, yet they never seemed to go away either. A new one had appeared and I felt concerned about this. It was during a meditation (with a women's group I belong to) that a startling piece of information came to me. I suddenly KNEW that what I was afraid of (in relation to my breast lumps) was not being sick, or having cancer, or even of dying. What really struck a cold fear in my gut was dealing with the medical world: doctors, hospitals, sterile rooms, invasive procedures. Specifically what terrified me was the feeling of having my body taken away from me, of being powerless at the hands of some impersonal doctor. The whole world of the AMA was where the real sickness was!!! I realized that I needed to be in charge of my health, my body, and my healing—not that I had to do it all by myself: having helpers is essential; but I had to be the one in charge. It was after all my body.

Then I got my checkup and the doctor strongly suggested I get a mammogram. I knew deep inside me that that felt wrong for me. That is when I called you, Ingrid, and learned about the salves.

Shortly after I realized that I was dealing with a serious healing crisis, I went to get a reading with a woman who is a psychic and (who) has been very helpful to me and my family for several years. The information from the guides was very helpful. And this one particular thing I want to share with you . . . the psychic said to me, "I notice that the guides are not using the word 'cancer'."

. . . They told me . . . not to call in that thoughtform. They said that the idea or word 'cancer' carries with it tremendous fear; it is a well developed thoughtform built from many hundreds of thousands of peoples' pain, suffering, dread, and confusion. To call it to myself would only be like calling in a terrible dark cloud over my head. This has been very useful information. While I do not wish to be in denial, I recognize I am dealing with a very serious condition. I continue to think of what I 'have' as a healing crisis. With the help of the salves, I am ridding my body of dead and useless matter.

From the very first time I used the salves, I felt like I was a witness to one of the Seven Wonders of the World!! It was like that. I just felt such awe, such appreciation to you, Ingrid, for making these salves

known, to the forces of Nature from which these salves are derived, to the Intelligence in the Universe. Every time I use the black salve and start another round, I feel like I am witness to a miracle. The scabs really form, crack, and fall off, just like the instructions say! It is such an incredible process. As of now, the original lumps that I had are gone. I felt one of the lumps dissolve under my very fingers over the span of 24 hours! It is truly an amazing thing . . . and to think the FDA would try to ban this!

Another thing which I noticed in myself during this time was somewhat surprising to me. Whenever the scabs formed and while they were cracking and falling off, I have never felt separate from them. I have never felt disgusted . . . Instead, it has always been more of a sense that this matter, this "stuff" coming out of me is ME. It is mine. It is old me, and even dead me. I don't need it anymore and I know that definitely it is time for this "me" to come out and get flushed away. I am not afraid of it. I'll tell you, it has been shocking to notice this. It is not what I expected I would feel. Somehow when these scabs fall off, I hold them and feel such a sense of gratitude! That sounds astounding! I think so too—but that is the honest truth. Perhaps this dead "stuff" which comes out was trying to be useful to me in some way I can't understand. Whatever, I thank it as it passes out of me. It most certainly is time to build new parts of myself in a more Lighted way.

The most important and wonderful thing about this process for me has been that I feel like I am in charge of my own healing. I am the responsible one. I certainly feel you and Susan as tremendous support. It would be almost impossible to do this without you! But you haven't taken my power away, you don't try to control me. It's not like this is YOUR process which you are doing TO me. I am in charge—and I am profoundly happy about that! This is how it should be. And I should add, this escharotic treatment is truly not for the faint of heart. It is intense. When it is painful . . . it is really something. It's a mess: bandages, gooey salves. It doesn't make dealing with breast lumps a nice easy procedure. It is heavy duty, but it sure beats surgery! And in my book, it clearly beats dealing with the medical establishment.

All in all, it has been an amazing adventure and a most profound time of learning. There really are no words yet invented which could tell you how grateful I am to you, Ingrid. The work you do is truly earth-shaking.

/S.T./

Dear Ingrid and Susan,

Thank you for all of your tremendous work. I spoke with a woman last night who asked if I had seen you. I said, "No, but I feel as if I am in constant consultation through the tapes." The tapes give me information, but mainly I get energy by the sound of your voice, Ingrid, your tone, and the manner you deal with it all.

I am on my second round of the black salve. My tumor was hard and big as a baseball. It is going down. The changes are tremendous. It hurts. Yes, it hurts! but it is working! I feel the alchemy of it concentrate my whole being. I feel something inside of me being magnetized to the Earth. I have a vision of the Black Madonna reaching her hand out from the inner core of the Earth and saying, "Stay here. This is where you need to be—united with the deep core of Earth."

The cancer feels to be my negativity drawn up together, so that I can get rid of it. I feel myself mutating. I can feel the darkness drawing in tremendous light. I've had two dreams connected with the golden salve, one dancing in a golden dress, and one wearing a golden cape.

I want to be in further communication with you.

Bless you!

/S.L./

Dear Ingrid,

I have been meaning to tell you that the "herbal bullets" have cleared up a chronic vaginal condition I thought I had to live with forever. I am deeply grateful!

/H.R./

Dear Ingrid,

Since using the goldenseal ointment, not only has my tumor regressed but my whole being has begun to feel healthier and more alert.

/R.W./

"S.T." is very much alive and well. She followed her inner guidance and sought only a minimal amount of medical advice and has had no recurrence since using the salves in 1991.

"S.L." tried eight different cancer treatments before her incredible rendezvous with fate. A video was made before her death. She shared her process with the depth of a true seeker. In a certain way, Sara is still very much alive. She has transmitted volumes from the Beyond to her husband, Elias Lonsdale. *The Book of Theanna* is a passionate tale of her spiritual destiny and the healing that is necessary for this Planet—and how it is being assisted from the Invisible Realms. I have often felt her presence while working on this manuscript.

"H.R." used the suppositories and is well today.

"R.W." is alive and continues to make improvement.

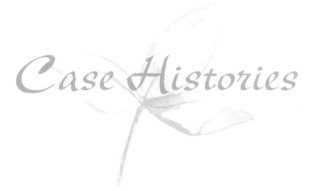

CHAPTER 6

Case Histories

As previously noted, very few of the many stories related to me by lay practitioners were supported by proper diagnostic tests that confirmed the existence of cancer. Even fewer were accompanied by long-term follow up. However, as might be expected, physicians tended to keep better records. First among these was Mr. Richard Guy, a London surgeon who, in 1759, published a paper describing one hundred cases treated by a poultice whose formula was not divulged. A century later, Dr. J. Weldon Fell's work was peer reviewed. The findings as well as a description of the paste and his methodology were published. Dr. John Pattison, a contemporary of Fell, also published a detailed description of his enucleating paste and adjunctive cancer treatments; and, approximately fifty years later, Dr. Eli G. Jones published case histories along with the particular protocols used on the patients under his care. By the time Jones published his book, he had treated over 20,000 patients. Finally, two centuries after Guy, Frederic E. Mohs of the

University of Wisconsin Medical School published a book in 1956 entitled *Chemosurgery in cancer, gangrene and infections*.[47] Mohs delayed publication of *Chemosurgery* for five years in order to permit adequate evaluation of the technique he used. When he went to press, he had used the *fixed tissue technique*, with five-year results, in 9,716 cases of basal cell carcinoma and 3,299 cases of squamous cell carcinoma of the skin.

Though Mohs emphasizes the use of his technique with skin cancers, he discusses treatment of other "accessible structures" of the body as well as infections and gangrene. This is consistent with all uses of the salve by lay and professional practitioners alike. Mohs provided photographs of before-and-after pictures of sites treated as well as statistics dealing with the success rate for tumors treated at various stages of malignancy. In some instances, he had follow-up data spanning twenty-two years of treatment. This is certainly the most professional presentation of data on salve use, but the entire book deals with a single technique applied to a variety of tumors in more or less the same manner.

I cite this book mainly for the record and for the benefit of physicians and skeptics who may wish to study it. Mohs and Hoxsey used the same, or at least a nearly identical, escharotic paste. However, the Mohs method and reporting differed significantly from that of his controversial contemporary. His work meets the demands of science for proofs. Nevertheless, even today, Hoxsey is better known by the public, partly because he had the largest chain of cancer hospitals in history—and partly, no doubt, because he attracted press, even long after his death.

When the film "Hoxsey: How Healing Becomes a Crime,"[48] produced by Ken Ausubel and Catherine Salveson, was premiered in Santa Fe, I happened to be seated next to a woman who had been treated at the Hoxsey Clinic twenty years previously. During the intermission, she related her story to me and maintained that she has been in continuous good health since her treatment. It is my understanding that, for a flat one-time fee, it was, at one time, the policy of the Hoxsey Clinic to provide Hoxsey *graduates* with annual supplies of the internal tonic for the rest of their lives. I am quite certain that this makes a difference in terms of recurrence since the salves are a substitute for surgery—not a lifetime guarantee of freedom from cancer.

Well-documented, clear case histories are valuable, but they are also scarce. In the pages that follow, a few examples of proven cures that relied on escharotics are provided. The first comes from Hoxsey, and it is one of the more dramatic in the annals of escharotic history.

PATIENT OF HOXSEY TREATMENT, MUSCATINE, ILLINOIS, 1930[49]

One of the earliest and most spectacular cases treated during this period was Mandus Johnson of Galesburg, Illinois. When I first saw him on March 2, 1930, the entire top of his head was covered with a cancer (the biopsy had been made by a Dr. Baird of Galesburg). It had consumed the entire scalp, exposing the skull. Two drain tubes had been inserted into holes cut in the skull, and from these more than a pint of pus was drained every day. To this day it remains the worst case of cancer I have ever seen.

"Either cure me or kill me!" he begged. "I can't stand the odor, I'd rather be dead than like this." I had to tell him there wasn't but one chance in a million that he would survive. However I agreed to try.

Five weeks later I went on the radio and announced that the following night (April 8th) we would remove the top of Johnson's skull, and the cancer with it. People came as far as 800 miles to witness the operation. When Dr. Rasmussen and I lifted the cancer from the sick man's head, exposing the brain, 14 people in the audience fainted.

The AMA Journal immediately published a vicious attack upon us, asserting that Johnson had died as the result of our treatment. We quickly spiked that lie. On Decoration Day (May 30th) the "dead man" made a personal appearance—with over 100 other patients—at a giant demonstration in Weed Park, Muscatine.

METASTATIC CANCER

This next story is apt to evoke agonizing echoes in many others. At the time we met, this woman had been given only weeks to live. Though she appeared to be following our discussion, the logic had failed to register. She apparently grasped the gist of the conversation but none of the details.

When in her late thirties, this woman found a tumor in her right breast. She had a mastectomy in which all of the lymph nodes were removed. She then underwent three months of chemotherapy. Because the tumor was estrogen sensitive, five months after the mastectomy, she had a total hysterectomy. This was followed by reconstructive surgery of the right breast along with the recommendation that her left breast be reduced to match the reconstructed right one. It was after all this that she developed an interest in alternative medicine, attended a school of natural medicine for a year, and learned of some new approaches she hoped would help her.

About four years after the original treatment of the breast cancer, she became severely dyslexic and eventually was unable to make herself understood by others. Tests revealed that she had metastatic brain tumors. As her letter that follows states, she refused brain surgery. She was told she had two months to live. She had a single treatment with stereotaxic radio therapy, 27 and 29 rads pinpointed on the two tumors. Immediately following this treatment, she applied the black salve to her neck at the base of the skull. She ran a systemic fever following the first application of a bloodroot paste.[50] This was followed by use of the yellow healing salve. She made a full recovery. I asked her to what she attributed her remarkable rally. I specifically requested that she check with the radiologist (who knew she intended to begin use of the salve after the radiation treatment) in order to get a solid opinion on the medical aspects of her regression. Both she and her doctor attributed the destruction of the tumor and its disappearance more to the salves than to the radiation, which was reportedly only able to destroy the centers of the tumors. The opening on her neck was quite large, probably twice what would have sufficed in her situation, and the amount of exudation from the opening was substantial. However, she reported that, aside from the first few nights, she felt "great" while using the salves, that she was able to return to work, and that she had gained a renewed faith in her future. Magnetic resonance imaging (MRI) showed that the mass shrank considerably after five to six weeks on the salves, and even more after three months. Routine MRIs that were performed considerably later revealed a slight amount of scar tissue but no malignancy. The pictures taken by magnetic resonance imaging are hers. As can be seen, there was a significant reduction of both the tumor and the edema following application of the salve.

Excerpts from her letter written in early 1992 follow:

The salves gave me new hope. I had been diagnosed with two metastatic brain tumors. The treatments offered were unacceptable to me. One was full brain radiation, and the second was open brain surgery to remove one of the tumors.[51] To me, both treatments were worse than the disease.

. . . New hope flooded me the moment I heard about the salves. Here was something I could actively participate in to remove the tumors. I felt control coming back in my life. I also had a positive outlook again.

The twenty-four hours with the black salve were painful. I could still go about my daily routine, but I had a fever the first three nights of the treatment. I considered the fever an added bonus as higher body temperatures can kill cancer cells.

It took about three weeks for the yellow salve to stop draining out any more yellowish-green material. I put the black salve on again and only a small lesion appeared. I waited until the hole completely healed this time. When I put the black salve on the third time, nothing happened.

The scar is not bad and I rub Weleda Arnica Massage oil into it two times a day. It is smoothing out nicely.

She was right about the fever. The importance of temperature to cancer was accidentally discovered when Dr. William B. Coley, a nineteenth century New York surgeon, began searching for the key to why some patients died soon after surgery for cancer while others seemed cured. The answer was not what a researcher might have expected: those who recovered had contracted infections while hospitalized and ran fevers. To date, I have not seen concurrence as to the temperature needed to destroy cancer cells, but Dr. Robert Atkins suggests that cancer dies when the temperature reaches 104°–105.8°F (see page 43).

Though Coley's findings have prompted others to experiment with deliberately induced bacterial infections, it seems that the pharaohs and Hippocrates already knew the relationship of heat to cancer. In the natural health community, hyperthermia treatments and toxic herbs have been used to raise temperatures. Not all patients respond to toxins by running fevers, but when they do, the results have often been quite positive. In any event, fever may have played a role in the short-term recovery just cited.

More than a year later there was a recurrence. This time she did not use the salves. Initially, she sought relief in new spiritual practices. Eventually, when suffering from six tumors in the brain, she submitted to four craniotomies. She did not recover from this struggle.

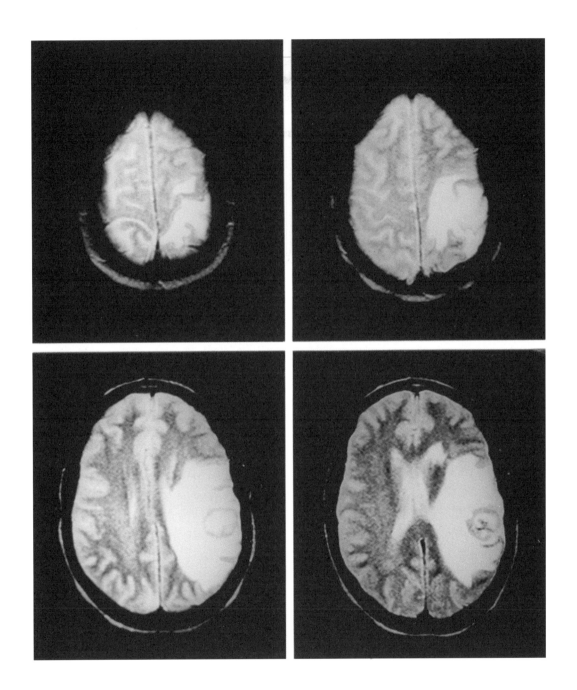

M.R.I.
October 2, 1991

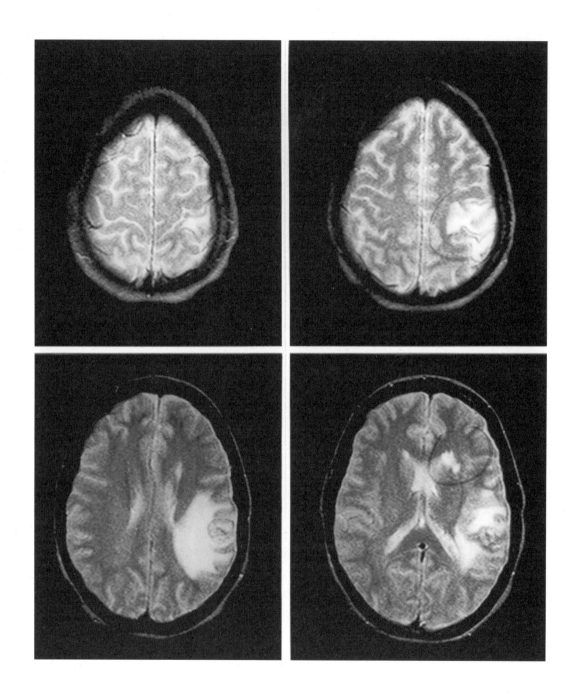

M.R.I.

January 2, 1992

Less than two months after beginning use of the salve.

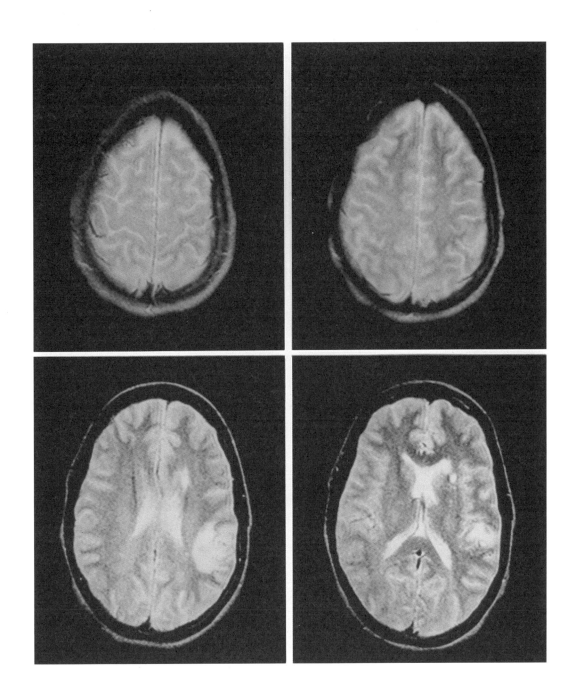

M.R.I.

March 3, 1992

After discontinuing use of the salve.

QUALITY OF LIFE

My own relationship to the salves is inseparable from the tale of Susan Meares. In the spring of 1990, she was told that she had an inoperable form of cancer and, at most, a year to live. She was offered an experimental form of chemotherapy. She believed "experimental" was a euphemism for "even more horrible than the conventional cytotoxic protocols." She left the hospital and went straight to a bookstore. There she found a book on diet by a Dutch doctor named Moerman. This was the beginning of a major quest for an alternative cure for cancer.

Susan and I met in August of that year. She had just turned forty-six. She was enterprising and incredibly disciplined. I listened as she described her situation and her life, and I loaned her some books and video tapes that I thought might enhance her meager education on alternatives. Among these was the film about the work of Harry Hoxsey as well as some ghastly video footage taken by the family of a patient in New Jersey who had used the salve on a metastatic condition in the liver. The patient's screaming was painfully audible on the video, and I told Susan that the woman had died. However, according to the family, an autopsy had been done and no cancer had been found. At the time, I did not really understand what had happened. I knew that there had been a crisis with another member of the family and that the woman had gone off her careful diet, swelled up with bloating, been given morphine for the pain, and died in a hospital some days later; but this is all the information I had.

All I knew that I could, at that time, relay to Susan was that someone who was using the salve for nasal polyps had gone to a local herb shop and told the employees there what he was doing. The way the story was told to me was that the salve he was using was an old Native American formula passed on from the grandfather to the man who was making it. At this juncture, I am not certain that the details imparted at that time were entirely accurate; however, as you can see, I was spurred to keep asking questions.

Susan decided to try the salves. Her tumor was enormous, about four by twelve inches, and it extended from the sternum to the armpit. Susan believed she had created a shield over her heart to protect herself from pain; but she was, at least in the beginning of her illness, determined to survive. The salves were a nuisance, and, like many people, she had a love-hate relationship with them. Still, she felt quite positive about her response to them, and they seemed to be her best bet. If the instructions for their use had been more reliable, who knows what the outcome might have been. Susan used the salves for seven months and became an expert on bandaging. In the spring of 1991, when she was supposed to be dead, she had a somewhat experimental blood test for cancer, the CA 15-3, which was two points above normal. A year later, she repeated the test; the results of this one were completely normal. Since only months after our first meeting, Susan had been working for me. Seeing her interest in dietary approaches to cancer treatment, I had hired her to help research a nutritional guide for people with cancer. Thus, for the last years of Susan's life, I saw her practically every day.

In the summer of 1992, for reasons perhaps known only to her, she told me that she did not believe cancer to be curable, and she gave up the effort to save her life. For many months, she seemed to be on a plateau. I was concerned that, in the long run, the plateau was not a safe place; but I could also see that she was making her own decisions. She felt good; there was no immediate danger. She was enjoying life—she even took up snorkeling.

Susan had two years of remarkable health. She had some burning sensations on the black salve days; but, otherwise, she enjoyed a normal life. She had taken many internal tonics and was, according to outer appearances as well as the blood tests, in good shape. However, she stopped taking the very supplements that had made such a difference during the two years following the original diagnosis. After that turning point, nothing motivated her to defy the odds.

The plateau lasted a long time. It was nine months, March 1993, before she had the first minor symptom: a little pain in her shoulder that was relieved by two Advils™. She refused to consult any doctors. Another few months passed before the extent of the hidden problems became evident. By July, she had problems with coordination and speech. She went on a vacation with her family, had an MRI, and discovered she had a brain tumor and very little time to live. I last saw her on her forty-ninth birthday, July 23. At that time, she was still able to hike, but her speech was labored.

Compared to patients who spend months or years of their lives bedridden or on pain relievers such as morphine, the quality of Susan's life was extraordinary. If holistic medicine has nothing else to offer, at least it does not compromise the quality of life. Susan died on August 14, 1993. I gave up my fascination with the salves and brooded on fate. It has taken me almost three years to pick up where I left off—and I definitely wish that the information in this book had been available in 1990.

SUCCESSFUL TUMOR REMOVAL

At about the same time that Susan was using the black and yellow salves, I knew several other people using the same salves. Many of them are today completely well, more than seven years after starting their use of escharotic treatment; many had no recurrence or complications beyond modest scarring. These conditions included breast tumors, melanomas, and Kaposi's sarcoma lesions.

Also, because my investigation of the salves has been noted in several books by other authors, my telephone rings constantly with "salve stories." They are all anecdotal, and I seldom ask for medical records because I feel that this is the job of those who pick up the gauntlet and research the salves properly. However, the few stories that follow are worth relating.

A woman who formerly owned a health foods store used the salves to treat a large mass on her arm. She is completely healed and well. An acupuncturist took the escharotics internally for cancer of the tongue. He spit out two tumors while sitting across from me at my desk. They were the size of peas, and the sight was unforgettable. One man with sarcoma in the ears discharged six tumors of varying dimensions, half an inch to an inch, using only an escharotic salve. A group of orthodox Jewish people in New York is using the black and yellow salves as a matter of religious and medical choice. The husband of the person who makes these particular salves had liver cancer in 1977 and continues to be fine today. The mother of the maker of one of the Compound X formulae used that paste at the age of seventy-five when she developed a large tumor near the clavicle. She is now ninety-four years old and in excellent health except for a little itching around the scar tissue. This salve is being used by Buddhist monks of the Shao Lin Temple in China.

LAWYER

A lawyer whose breast cancer had been treated conventionally became dissatisfied with conventional treatments and began searching for alternatives. Being resourceful, she managed to track me down through people she was certain would know me. She told me that she had an escharotic salve and wondered if it were safe to use. After telling her what I knew, she applied it to her leg. She called to tell me that much was being discharged through the hole created by the salve: "I really see it working—it's just amazing!"

MEDICAL DOCTOR WITH RECURRENCE

A doctor in her early thirties had a mammogram that revealed lumps, one in each breast. One was surgically biopsied and the other surgically excised, leaving a gaping hole. Sometime thereafter, she had a hysterectomy because of uterine fibroids and bleeding. Nearly a decade later, she noticed blood on her nightgown; she was afraid, went into denial, but recognized that her nipples were retracted. Another physician sent some of the blood for testing: atypical cells were found. At the time, both doctors had taken their first steps into holistic medicine, mainly homeopathy. The patient was determined not to have any more surgery on her body.

She was acquainted with a shaman who had himself been using the "black salve" on an obscure growth. She decided to try the salve and used it according to the directions provided: once a week. Though she sometimes used Motrin™ for pain, the breast was at times so painful that she could not even stand the jostling when her car went over a bump in the road, but she persevered for seven weeks until the area seemed clean. She was really surprised by the way the crater healed; in just a few days, it filled in remarkably, though she lost a bit of the areola around the nipple. This treatment was complete more than three years ago, and she has had no further indications of recurrence.

When asked how she felt about the salve, she said that if friends consulted her and expressed sufficient determination to avoid surgery, she would discuss the salve with them.

FAITH

For me, the treatments offered by conventional medicine are too abhorrent to consider. I have often asked myself what it would be like to be in the patient's shoes, to have the same fears the patient has, and to be confronted with the same decisions a patient has to make.

I suppose I asked myself this question once too often because in the spring of 1994, a lump the size of a walnut appeared on my rib cage. It had the classic appearance of a malignancy. I knew exactly what would happen if I went to a doctor: biopsies, recommendations presented more in the form of ultimata than suggestions, lectures about being sensible and allowing him or her to do what he or she knows to be right, invasive procedures, pain, and so forth. This occurred at an intensely busy time in my life; I hardly had space to think, but after brooding for a few days, I ran for the salve and the psychics. In the first nearly sleepless night (using Dr. Christopher's cayenne salve, *Red Sun Balm*), I relived nearly every story I had ever heard from patients with cancer. I felt their pain, even their quiet heroism.

Fortunately for me, the salve worked very quickly; and, as it happened, by the end of the second day on the salve, the upper part (the part that had looked so foreboding) fell off, and what remained had the appearance of a sebaceous cyst rather than a malignancy. Anyway, I got to try out the shoes I had never worn before, and I discovered that I would, in fact, trust my own well-being to the salves. However, I emphasize that I consulted a very competent channel to inquire as to the deeper symbolism of the development. I got an answer that made perfect sense to me, and an immediate body-mind connection was formed that enabled me to work consciously with a process that I knew had deep significance for me. I also took a look at my overall health and devoted myself to making some improvements

BEFORE CONTINUING

It is very important for me as the person reporting on this method of cancer treatment that the information I impart is both accurate and well focused. In the Preface, I tried to establish the fact that I am principally a medical philosopher, a theorist rather than a practitioner. Moreover, I am inclined to take such a broad view of the disease process that I might be guilty of ignoring pathology in favor of psychology. My own experience supports the safety of this bias, but I do not think it is safe to ignore any challenge that occurs in life. Therefore, I have continually emphasized the need for an intelligent relationship to what is happening physically and emotionally. Neither passivity nor ignorance nurture the inner being who is frightened, bewildered, and often angry about what is happening. Thus, to put a proper perspective on this report on escharotics, I must emphasize that though I personally believe that the herbal approaches to cancer treatment are valuable, I do not regard them as a complete response to a life threatening disease such as cancer.

Cure, in my estimation, entails shifting the cause that underlies the symptoms and pathologies. It means finding out what is really wrong and correcting the problems at their source. It means making a commitment to wellness that involves the whole being, not hoping for a shortcut or quick answer that will put one back on the fast track again. This said, I invite you to explore the next section of the book; it contains the instructions for use of the escharotic products.

However, before going on, I would like to reiterate my opinion that a life threatening illness, however responsive to treatment it might be, should be viewed as more than a medical crisis. It is a challenge to life itself, and this challenge is best met by an assessment of the values guiding life and its priorities, by a serious effort to instill deep meaning into the life, and by whatever changes in life style and attitude the answers to the challenges to life dictate.

PART THREE

The Methods

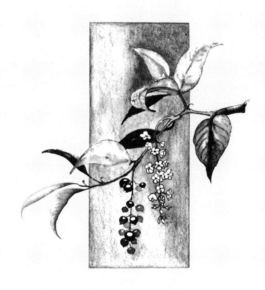

POKE
Phytolacca decandra

*T*HE NEXT THREE CHAPTERS *contain instructions for use of the escharotic products. Health care professionals will want to study the various methods carefully so as to acquire insights into the nuances of treatment. Patients are advised to read chapters VII and VIII for generalities and to study chapter IX thoroughly before commencing use of any product similar to those described in this book. The decision to use the salve as well as the consequences of such choice are, of course, entirely those of the patient.*

CHAPTER 7

Pattison Method

1866

$\mathcal{I}$N MY RESEARCHES OF THE HISTORIC USES of escharotics and of the persons who used them, four figures stood out as exceptional.

•Hildegard of Bingen was the first. Her recipes and visions survived, but we know little of her methodology and nothing of her cure rate.

•John Pattison, M.D., 1866, was the next. He is a personal favorite because of his exceptional gentility and clarity. He believed enucleation to be superior to other treatments for cancer because the method is founded on common sense. His writing was superb and his modesty touching. His eclecticism stretched my understanding of constitutional responsiveness to treatment; his success remains unrivaled; and his methodology was disclosed in considerable detail. I have therefore chosen to present a relatively thorough overview of his protocols.

•I will do the same with respect to the work of Dr. Eli Jones, the third individual, whose protocols were more elaborate and every bit as eclectic as those of Pattison. Though his books have been reprinted in India and are available worldwide, including from the Seventh Ray Press, they merit summarization here. This has been done in the next chapter.

Dr. John Christopher is the fourth on my list. His writing was extensive and is readily available in print as well as on CD-ROM, thereby obviating the need to cover it in as much detail as his predecessors. It should however be noted that Christopher's cancer treatments have been distilled in *The Layman's Course on Killing* Cancer by Sam Biser and later by his brother Loren Biser. This latter is planned for release in a CD-ROM version. There are also video tapes of the work of Dr. Richard Schulze, a student of Christopher's, who continues to work with protocols for "incurables" similar to those of his teacher.

Before presenting the instructions on the use of the escharotics, the subject of this and the next two chapters, I wish to interject a few personal notes.

The process that has brought me to the point where I could pull together the material for this book has been long, revelatory, and emotionally strenuous. I listened to the suffering and occasionally to the excitement of patients while also coming to grips with the truly shocking history of Western medicine. How Christians who rejoiced in the tales of the healings of Jesus could withhold relief from their brethren has been perplexing. How they could murder so many natural healers and women in the name of God is beyond comprehension. It simply defies reason. It would be pointless to remind society of these atrocities unless modern medicine were at least in some respects a direct descendent of this pseudo-Christian and pseudo-scientific era. I personally do not believe that conventional medicine has extricated itself from the darker motivations of its predecessors: control of information with the objective of economic domination. Until it is able to clean its own house and police its own work, it will remain unreliable.

My purpose is not to accuse anyone, merely to fault the system enough to empower individuals to look beyond the system for hope. If the system were willing to question itself by critically assessing its reasons for failure, it would deserve the grants and monopolies it currently enjoys. However, the fact that it performs almost no reasonable outcome studies suggests that its monopoly is a matter of money and politics rather than merit.

CURE FOR CANCER

Many are looking for a cure for cancer. Some are reinventing the wheel by performing variations of studies already carried out ad nauseam, such as more investigations into carcinogens or possible viral links to cancer. Others are synthesizing substances that can be patented, testing them on innocent mice whose tumors do not develop spontaneously but rather are transplanted into them. The argument that a cure for human cancers may be found by subjecting animals to inhumane experiments is probably sincerely believed but spurious. Science is not even capable of questioning whether the shrinkage of tumors is due to drugs or inherent vitality and immune response or separation of healthy cells from malignant ones. These issues vex me. Therefore, a voice of reason, even if from an earlier era, is refreshing.

Pattison's grounded approach to treatment is almost unparalleled in today's world. He saw patients in his private consulting rooms, conversed with them every day, and observed their responses first hand rather than on a printout from a person with whom he had never spoken. He maintained a proper equilibrium between compassion and technicality and remained alert to the fact that people have cancer and doctors are merely the agents of hope and relief.

I disclaim all claims to infallibility, for in such a scourge, we can only hope for radical cures in comparatively few cases, but expect to afford relief to all. Indeed, however simple the case may be that comes before me, in no one instance have I ever promised to effect a cure, for I am only an instrument in God's hands, who, without His blessing, would toil to cure, or relieve, in vain.[52]

We recall that it was Pattison who introduced the use of American herbal alkaloids to his British colleagues. It was also Pattison who challenged the allopathic use of caustics, such as the arsenic based preparations that were popularized in England by Justamond in the Seventeenth Century and in France a century later by Girouard. Pattison especially disliked the treatments based on pure zinc chloride because of the intolerable pain. He faulted Fell for his use of zinc chloride even though Fell's success rate was also remarkable for his day. Pattison felt that zinc chloride may be more dangerous than surgery because of the damage it does to tissue structure. His blending of goldenseal with zinc chloride was based on trials that showed that goldenseal has specific effects on the disease that reduce pain and the risk of recurrence of the disease while increasing the effects of zinc chloride.[53]

Though Pattison's method was derived from those of Justamond and Girouard, his enucleating paste contained different agents and caused considerably less pain.[54] His paste was mildly irritating when applied to healthy tissue but more specific with regard to malignancy. Pattison's treatments go beyond what might be called modifications or refinements. He addressed the overall state of the patient, minimized pain, and maximized the selectivity of zinc chloride's destructive power. Together, these factors constituted a new approach to cancer treatment— though Pattison was not naïve enough to imagine that his protocols would be accepted by the medical profession, a profession he described as resistant to new ideas.

Pattison's Technique

Without writing fifty pages on the subject, it is difficult to do Pattison justice. It will be necessary, at times, to generalize in order to outline the basics of his method. First of all, Pattison made a distinction between tumors that are on the surface or that have ulcerated and those that are deeper. If the tumor was deep, he believed that caustics do more harm than good. To address such masses, he found it necessary to use a dilute solution of nitric acid before applying the escharotic, or as he called it "enucleating paste." He used only a few drops of the acid, specific gravity of 1.35, and rubbed it into the skin over the tumor. The area turned whitish by the following day. The procedure caused a few moments of discomfort, but the pain was not excruciating and subsided in ten to fifteen minutes. It is possible that Hoxsey's use of trichloroacetic acid was for a similar purpose. It, like zinc chloride, is a deliquescent crystal that is caustic in its own right that could have been used to break through the surface tissue.

For the first day, the nitric acid application was the only treatment. On the following day, Pattison applied an ointment that consisted of one part of his enucleating paste (equal parts of the powdered root of goldenseal, zinc chloride, flour, and water) and nine parts *calendula* (marigold) ointment. This created very little, if any, pain. Each day he increased the potency of ointment until the surface area was deadened, the nerves became numb and less sensitive, and feeling was lost. Then, by the end of the first week, he began making scratches in the eschar half an inch apart. He was careful never to cut deeper than the deadened area. He applied undiluted enucleating paste to tiny strips of linen and placed them in the cuts. These strips were only left in place for an hour or two, but the procedure was repeated daily until the tumor was completely destroyed. At this stage of the process, patients felt more discomfort than pain. However, many were feverish or sometimes restless at night. They also had some torpidity of the liver and bowels and loss of appetite. For fever, he administered homeopathic *Aconitum napellus* (monkshood) 2 or *Veratrum viride* (white American hellebore) 2. For appetite, he gave *Mercurius solubilis* 2 or *Leptandrine* (culver's root) 2. For biliary attacks, he gave two to four drops of *Veratrum album* (white hellebore) 2 or *Ipecacuanha* (ipecac root) 2. I am not a homeopath, but I looked up these remedies in the *Materia Medica*, and the usages described there were consistent with Pattison's prescriptions.

Gradually, the tumor died and began to feel heavy. When the tumor was completely destroyed, Pattison discontinued use of the strips with the enucleating paste. He did nothing for four to five days while the line of demarcation between the living and dead parts developed. He learned by experience to avoid ointments at this time because the viscosity retarded the separation process. As the eschar started to separate, he dressed strips of calico with calendula ointment and placed them around the eschar, one half overlaying the eschar, the other half overlapping the surrounding healthy tissue. He changed these once a day. By about the tenth day, the separation between the eschar and living tissue had widened significantly, finger width. He then discontinued use of the calico strips and used cotton wool medicated with the same calendula ointment. The tumor usually fell out between the fourteenth and twenty-first day following the removal of the dressings with the enucleating paste. The average was sixteen days, the shortest was twelve days, and the longest was thirty-three.

INSPECTION

In most cases, eschars detach without the patient noticing until the dressings are changed. Pattison wrote that once the mass detaches, a flat surface is exposed to view. It is covered with purulent matter but is bloodless. He dressed this area with calendula ointment. It is at this time that expert examination of the area for traces of remaining malignancy is necessary. Untrained persons may or may not be able to detect such residuals. Since the tumor is a different color from the healthy tissue, once the first eschar detaches, it is usually possible to determine whether the entire mass has been enucleated or whether parts of the tumor remain in the area. If any part remains, it is necessary to apply diluted enucleating paste to that spot. Pattison stated that only one in a hundred persons required additional treatment. In this regard, his method seems superior to that of others using escharotics.

Once the entire area is determined to be cancer free, the procedure varies considerably according to the practitioner. Pattison used *unguent resinosum flavæ* if the area exhibited a tendency to be indolent. He mixed this with one-eighth its weight of *spiritus terebinthini*. The next day, he dressed the area with powdered goldenseal and honey. Sometimes, he used cloths dipped in cold infusions of goldenseal; other times, he dressed the site with a lotion made from hot-water infusions of *Phytolacca decandra* (poke root). He varied these according to the appearance of the site: "No definite rule can be laid down as what to employ." The healing process took three to four weeks once the mass had detached.

Adjunctive Measures

During this healing period, Pattison began administering prophylactic remedies. He felt that it was these measures that established the fact that cancer is actually curable. To understand his opinion, it is necessary to compare the enucleating process with surgery.

Pattison regarded enucleation as a method of tumor removal, not a cure. The cure required more specific measures. He objected to the idea that tumors that appear to fluctuate do so because they contain fluids that can be removed via various external applications.

In the healing stage, Pattison used homeopathic remedies because he believed they reach where the grosser preparations do not. *Hydrastis canadensis* was his homeopathic remedy of choice. He said he used the first, third, sixth, or twelfth decimal dilutions. He gave the same remedy three to four times a day for a week. Then, he used resinous alkaloids such as *phytolaccin*, *cerasin*, and *heloniadine* in the second decimal dilutions, except for cerasin which he used in the mother tincture. He used *xanthoxylin* (from prickly ash) if the patient was weak, often alternating it with cerasin. He felt that these latter do not have the same anti-cancer effect as *hydrastin*, phytolaccin, and heloniadine, but their tonifying properties justified their use.

He recommended that certain of the treatments be continued for some months after the patient returned home. When these instructions were followed and *when stress to the affected area was carefully avoided*, he said there was no return of the disease.

Safety of the Method

Pattison summed up the description of his technique by emphasizing the safety of the method over surgery. Though he admitted to having made many mistakes early in his career, he said that he never lost a life through enucleation. He emphasized the need for experience, but stated that enucleation, when skillfully carried out, destroys the entire disease. Pattison said that surgeons are unable to view the diseased area completely because blood deluges the area. Therefore, when they close up, they are apt to leave some of the disease inside. However, with enucleation the mass detaches, leaving a clean and bloodless area. If any malignancy remains in this site, it is easily detected by an experienced practitioner. He maintained that these explanations account for why recurrence is more likely with surgery than enucleation.

Pattison described his method as relatively painless, saying that most patients did not lose sleep. Moreover, he felt that patients who were poor candidates for surgery, either because of their deterioration or nervous temperament, could be treated with his method. Patients who had recurrences after surgery described enucleation as far less painful than surgery. This said, Pattison admitted that his method is not infallible and that in a small number of cases the cancer does recur. He estimated recurrence rates to be approximately fifteen percent and stated that *imprudence on the part of the patient accounted for most of the recurrences.*

Pattison only used his enucleating method on about ten percent of patients. First of all, he saw the method as an aid, not a cure. The constitutional treatments were regarded as more important. The reasons he gave for using the enucleation method in so few cases were that people either presented themselves early enough that they could be cured by constitutional methods alone or that they came so late that there was little hope of effecting cure. However, even in these advanced states, he offered his constitutional remedies and certain topical applications in order to prolong life for a few months or years. He did not describe these protocols in detail, saying mainly that he needed to see the patient in person in order to have "a peculiar something" flash across his mind that dictated a certain treatment or medicine. When this instinctive feeling was absent, it seemed he was immobilized by uncertainty.

DIET

Pattison placed considerable emphasis on diet. In this, he was not alone, and he made nutrition a major part of his treatment. His first rule was that the patient needed nutritious food because deficiencies cause the disease to increase. He prohibited all food preserved by salt but insisted that food should be savory (salt that was added while cooking was evidently permitted).

To regulate the eliminatory system, he recommended fruits. When there was flatulence, he reduced the intake of vegetables. He suggested mild stimulants such as pale brandy and

PATTISON'S GOLDEN RULE

*Never irritate a malignant growth.
Always soothe it.*

"pure Hungarian wines," such as Carlowitz and Tokay, because of their phosphoric acid and iron contents and freedom from adulteration. In using such stimulants, he warned against depleting the vital power in any way.

As I found out when researching a book on diet for cancer patients, there is little consensus on this important subject. Recently, I suggested to a patient that she go abroad for treatment. The specialist running the clinic she visited recommended that all cancer patients eliminate fruit from their diets. He based this on the high sugar content of fruit; however, the grape cure is one of the regimes that I have occasionally seen to work—though it is very challenging. Also, contrary to the advice of Hildegard of Bingen, there are convincing studies attesting to the value of strawberries for breast cancer. Concurrence as to what constitutes a reasonable diet for persons with cancer seems unlikely in the near future.

PATTISON'S PRIMARY HERBS

Calendula officinalis, marigold, is a popular herbal medicine regarded by most botanists as mild and nontoxic. It is used to reduce infection and inflammation, remove toxins, decrease swelling, relieve lymphatic congestion, promote eruptions, and stimulate immunity. It is considered to be particularly effective in resolving tumors and cysts of the female reproductive system and breasts. It will be remembered that escharotic treatments were used predominantly on breast and skin

cancers so that practitioners had more experience with these types of cancer. Some modern sources warn that calendula should be used carefully with septic conditions because it promotes rapid healing.

Hydrastis canadensis, goldenseal, is one of the more highly regarded and expensive medicines in Nature's pharmacopoeia. It has many of the same properties as marigold in that it reduces infection and inflammation and stimulates immunity. It is also antimicrobial and can be used even in acute conditions. It, like calendula, is specific for tumors of the female reproductive system. By vitalizing the blood and reducing blood supply to tumors, its antitumoral effect is significant.

Though Pattison does not exactly explain his preference for these cooling herbs, it can be inferred from other of his statements that he opposed anything that might cause an increase of circulation to the affected area. For example, he advised against local heat applications because blood circulation will be greatest wherever the body is warmest. He saw this as a risk factor for metastasis. For the record, he also cautioned against the opposite: freezing. He said that with these methods, the initial pain is so agonizing that an inflammatory reaction occurs before the targeted part is frozen. His *golden rule* was, as noted, to keep the area as calm as possible. For this same reason, his method is the most gradual and apparently also the least painful of those I have been able to research.

Summary of the Pattison Method

1. Unless the tumor is near the surface or is ulcerated, rub the treatment area with a few drops of nitric acid of the specific gravity of 1.35. The surface should turn whitish.

2. On the following day, apply an ointment consisting of one part enucleating paste (equal parts of the powdered root of goldenseal, zinc chloride, flour, and water) and nine parts calendula ointment. This should create very little, if any, pain.

3. Increase the strength of the ointment each day (more enucleating paste) until, by the fifth or sixth day, the surface is thoroughly deadened and all feeling is lost.

4. With a very sharp implement, scratch the surface at half-inch intervals, being very careful not to cut deeper than the eschar.

5. Apply undiluted paste to thin strips of linen and place into cuts for an hour or two.

6. Continue with fresh dressings every day until the entire tumor is destroyed. As the procedure progresses, some discomfort is likely, but very little pain. The tumor will begin to feel heavy. Depending on the size and type of tumor, this process should not take more than four to five weeks.

7. When the tumor is destroyed, discontinue use of the strips with the enucleating paste.

8. Do not do anything for the next four or five days while the tumor is separating from the healthy tissue.

9. Dress strips of gauze with calendula ointment and place around the edge of the eschar, being certain that the strips overlap the living as well as the dead tissue. Change these once a day.

10. By the tenth day, it is usually possible to insert more deeply into the crack around the edge. Use cotton wool, medicated with the same calendula ointment, and insert into the crack around the edge. If the tumor is not completely destroyed, it will not separate properly.

11. The dead mass detaches as early as the twelfth day and as late as the thirty-third day, the norm being the sixteenth day.

12. *Never* try to hasten the removal.

13. After separation, a flat area covered with thick, purulent matter will be visible. It should be bloodless.

14. Dress this area with gauze spread with calendula ointment.

15. Repeat until the sore is cleansed. Examine visually for any trace of the tumor. If such is seen, dress the spot with the enucleating paste.

16. If the sore has a tendency to be indolent, dress with unguent resinosum flavæ mixed with 1/8 its weight of terebinthini.

17. Next day: dress with powdered goldenseal root mixed with honey; cloth dipped in cold infusion of goldenseal; or a lotion prepared from hot water infusion of poke root.

18. These applications vary according to the appearance of the sore.

19. The healing process is complete about three to four weeks after the mass has detached.

20. Begin prophylactic remedies.

For constitutional distress (feverishness, loss of appetite, restlessness at night, torpidity of the liver and bowels,) the following remedies were used by Pattison:

SYMPTOM	REMEDY
FEVER	Aconite 2 or Veratrum viride 2
LOSS OF APPETITE	Mercurius solubilis 2 or Leptandrine 2
OBSTINATE CONSTIPATION	Podophyllin or Leptandrine in 2-4 drop doses until the bowels are relieved
PAIN	1/4 to 1/3 grain codeine
RESTLESS AT NIGHT	Liquor nepenthe (made from morphia), 50-60 drops
SICKNESS, BILIARY ATTACKS	Veratrum album 2 or Ipecacuanha 2

GOLDENSEAL in homeopathic dilutions, 3rd, 6th, or 12th decimal; one dilution a week, three to four times daily, then interposing a week with resinous alkaloids, *phytolaccin, cerasin, heloniadine,* 2nd decimal solution, except cerasin which is used as mother tincture.

WEAK AND PROSTRATE, *xanthoxylin* alternating with *cerasin*. These have more of a tonic than anticancer effect.

These remedies are to be continued for some months after other treatments are completed. *Do not overexercise the affected side* of the body for some time.

Principal Agents used by Pattison

[Used both topically and internally.]

REMEDY	PART USED	INDICATIONS
Apocynin	root of *Apocynum cannabinum*	A cathartic and diuretic. For ovarian dropsy.
Asclepiadin	root of *Asclepias tuberosa*	An alterative, diuretic, and tonic. For peculiar rheumatic pains that are a frequent sequence of cancerous disease.
Atropin	leaves and roots of *Atropa belladonna*	Useful in neuralgia, fevers, especially those accompanied by eruptions, such as scarlet fever. Of benefit in mania, dependent on uterine disturbances.
Baptisin	stalks and leaves of *Baptisia tinctoria*	Valuable agent in treating amenorrhea. See also *Macrotidin*.
Caulophyllin	root of *Caulophyllum thalictroides*	For dysmenorrhea, leukorrhea, etc.
Cerasin	bark of *Cerasus virginiana*	Tonic. Can be given in place of quinine.
Collinsonin	root of *Collinsonia canadensis*	Influence on rectum and adjacent parts. Piles and abscesses.
Corydalidin	root of *Corydalis formosa*	Useful for scrofula.
Cyripedin	root of *Cyripedium pubescens*	Good tonic. Useful in chorea from its affinity to the purple lady slipper, *Sarcenia purpurea*. Useful in treating smallpox and similar exanthematous diseases.
Digitalidin	leaves of *Digitalia purpurea*	Rheumatism and cases where abortion is threatened.
Gelseminin	root of *Gelsemium sempervirens*	Excellent febrifuge, useful in rheumatic and neuralgic pains peculiar to cancerous growths.

REMEDY	PART USED	INDICATIONS
GERANIN	root of *Geranium maculatum*	Astringent. For hemorrhages and leukorrhea.
HAMAMELIDIN	leaves of *Hamamelis virginica*	Astringent and sedative. One of the most valuable agents in uterine disease.
HYDRASTIDIN	root of *Hydrastis canadensis*	Peculiar action on the mucous surfaces. Useful in cancerous affections of the liver or stomach, piles, leukorrhea, gonorrhea, otorrhea, etc.
LEPTANDRIN	root of *Leptandria virginica*	Gentle laxative, useful in treatment of piles, dyspepsia.
MACROTIDIN	root of *Macrotis racemosa*	See *Baptisin*.
MYRICIN	bark of the root of *Myrica cerifera*	Alterative and stimulant. Use when low state of body exists.
PHYTOLACCIN	root of *Phytolacca decandra*	Glandular affections.
PODOPHYLLIN	root of *Podophyllin peltatum*	Valuable cathartic, exerting a special influence on hepatic circulation.
SCUTELLARIN	*Scutellaria lateriflora*	Excellent tonic and antispasmodic. Useful in hysteria and nervous debility.
SENECIONIN	stalk and leaves *Senecio gracilis*	Diuretic and tonic. Useful in dropsy, debility, loss of appetite.
STILLINGIN	root of *Stillingia sylvatica*	Alterative and stimulant, useful in cutaneous diseases.
VERATRUM VIRIDE	concentrated tincture	Erysipelas. Paint the inflamed surface 3-4 times daily to prevent pitting. Mix with hydrastis.
VIBURNIN	bark of *Viburnum opulus*	Antispasmodic, alternative, and tonic. Useful in convulsions and threatened abortions.
XANTHOXYLIN	bark of *Xanthoxylum fraxineum*	Rheumatism and scrofula.

CHAPTER 8

Dr. Eli G. Jones

1911

*J*ONES HAD FOUR DECADES OF EXPERIENCE treating cancer before he committed his wisdom to words for the benefit of his successors. He said, "The successful treatment of cancer is the study of a lifetime and should not be attempted by a lazy man . . . ."[55] Writing at the beginning of this century, he bemoaned the loss of life by those who had surgery who "could have been saved by proper medical treatment."[56]

Jones believed that surgery is a shock to the nervous system that takes a major toll on the patient and results in lowered resistance to disease. He also felt that surgeons are unable to affect in any way the millions of cancer cells that circulate in the blood and constitute the origin of future tumors.

Jones was convinced that cancer results mainly from deterioration of the blood and debilitation or loss of vitality due to stress on the nerves. He cited poor eating and drinking habits as well as vaccinations as the primary causes of the corruption of the blood. He prescribed homeopathic *Thuja* 30X for "blood poisoning caused by vaccinations." If his charges of affluence and medical abuse sound familiar, it might be prudent to ask if anything really has changed for the better.

Jones treated cancer as a constitutional or blood disease and said, "It has been the hardest work of my life to make some doctors realize that the growth they see is only the effect, and that back of that lies the cause; and the cause must be removed before we can cure the cancer."

Jones was a cancer specialist who felt that cancer treatment demands that the physician have more skill than that required of any other specialist. He differentiated various types of cancers and maintained that what works for one type will have no effect on other types of cancer. Of those who sought his services, most, about four-fifths, had already undergone other treatments and suffered a recurrence worse than the original cancer. He claimed that of those who came to him first, before undergoing any other treatment, he was able to cure 95 percent—*permanently*—and that his patients remained cancer free for fifteen or twenty-five years.

He also noted that the complications—diabetes, heart disease, neuralgia, and such—drain the vitality of the patient. Jones used the term "nerve power" to measure the strength an individual has to resist disease and recover from it. Wars, financial stress, and anything else that causes worry, including the fears surrounding cancer itself, weaken nerve power and make the patient more susceptible to all diseases. His language differs from specialists today, but he was clearly describing the same factors that today are regarded as undermining to the body's immune system, but he described the stressors as depleting to the nerve power. Added to the list of external stressors were dietary indiscretions: excess consumption of tea, coffee, and meat.

Given his views, it is not surprising that Jones regarded the search for potent cytotoxic drugs as misguided. In his opinion, a poisonous drug would simply weaken the vitality of the patient and hasten his or her death. He cited five major causes of the rapid increase in the incidence of cancer in the civilized world:

Worry

Diminished nerve power opens the way for cancer. "In all countries where you find insanity on the increase, you will find cancer a close second. In Chicago, where insanity has increased the fastest in the world, cancer has increased 812% from 1861 to the present time (1911)." [57]

Vaccination

Jones found that the incidence of cancer was higher where there was enforced vaccination.

Meat-eating

He examined global statistics and noted that countries where meat consumption was low or vegetarianism was predominant, there were far fewer cases of cancer. "In the monastery of Grande Trappe, where the diet excludes tea, coffee, and meat, there has not been a case of cancer for twenty-seven years." [58]

Tea and coffee

Tea and coffee weaken the coats of the stomach and the nervous system. Jones related this to dyspepsia or indigestion. "In America, we are becoming a Nation of nervous, hysterical people, and insanity is on the increase." [59]

Alcoholic stimulants

"Good pure water, good pure air helps to make good healthy red blood. "

Jones stressed the need to teach people how to live. Cure depends first of all on the nerve power (or vitality) and secondly on whether or not the patient's system will respond to the remedies.

SURGERY AND RADIATION

Writing in 1911, Dr. Eli G. Jones remarked that for two hundred years, the medical profession had considered cancer to be a local disease. He personally felt that 95 percent of those who died might have been saved had they sought his services instead of those of surgeons. Jones traced this belief to the early founders of the Botanic School of Medicine one hundred years earlier, i.e., around the time of Rafinesque. When treating his first cancer patient in 1869, Jones became persuaded of the correctness of this theory. He had treated the patient for a blood disease, and the patient was cured. To emphasize his point, he cited countless studies noting that after surgery, cancer returns, often in less than half a year.[60] When it returns, it is, as Walshe said, more virulent than it had been before surgery. Jones thought this was partially explained by the trauma of the surgery to the patient's vitality. Jones used strong language: "To cut out a cancer is the worst form of malpractice, for it is only trying to remove the effect without touching the cause."[61]

The Eclectic School

Jones attended both Dartmouth Medical College and the Eclectic Medical College. It was in the latter that he was trained in the treatment and cure of cancer. Eclectic physicians were, according to Jones, the pioneers in the successful treatment of cancer. The belief that was widely held in the 1800s was that if the patient had basic constitutional strength, cure was probable through use of remedies that have definite remedial action upon abnormal conditions. For the cancer to regress, the general health had to be improved. This began with digestion, for healthy blood was believed to be dependent upon good digestion. Jones maintained that after forty-three years of spe-

cialization in the treatment of cancer, he was even more convinced that cancer can be cured: he was successfully treating 80 percent of those who came to him. He attributed the results mainly to his determination to treat the cancer as a local manifestation of a constitutional disease.[62]

Alcohol and Drugs

Jones stated that alcohol heats the blood and "acts the same on cancer as kerosene does on fire."[63] He advised avoiding treating substance abusers. He also stated that those who use drugs such as morphine and opium cannot be cured because the drugs work against the remedies needed to heal the patient. They also dry up secretions and weaken vitality.[64]

Since good digestion is required to make good blood, Jones paid attention to the digestion of each patient. If the digestion was poor, he treated this condition before considering the local treatments. In many ways, his pulse and tongue diagnostic methods sound more Ayurvedic than Western. His treatment began with the restoration of vitality and reduction of worry, for he viewed these as significant drains upon the all important nerve power. The more surgery a patient had had, the more the shock to the nervous system and the more important the remedies for restoring the strength of the nervous system. For this as well as injury from irradiation, he often used strychnine sulphate.

HOMEOPATHY

The basis of the Eclectic Medical tenets were that physicians should employ whatever methods and remedies work. As such, many doctors combined botanical medicine with homeopathy and other systems of healing that had shown results. Jones cited Drs. Edwin M. Hale, Richard Hughes, and J. Compton Burnett for their work in treating cancer homeopathically. In treating cancer with internal remedies, Jones relied heavily on the work of the British Burnett, author of a book describing 132 cures of breast cancer using homeopathy.

RECOMMENDATIONS

Though Jones was opposed to strong tea and coffee, he was not a "diet crank." He merely advised patients to chew their food well and to eat only what they can digest and assimilate. He noted that poor digestion can be determined by the color and coating of the tongue and that poor elimination is typical of patients in advanced stages of the disease.

One of his important recommendations was that patients take a bath in epsom salts at least twice a week. He suggested putting one pound of the salts into a tub of warm water and rubbing the skin until it is "as soft as velvet."[65] Believing as he did that cancer is mainly a disease of the blood, he said that the blood needs the magnesium in the epsom salts. In addition, he maintained that the epsom salts neutralize toxins in the blood, soothe tired

nerves, and help the patient "to rest like a tired child upon its mother's bosom."[66] He said that his treatments drive refuse matter to the surface and the epsom salts are necessary for cleansing.[67]

Jones believed that it is important to build up the general health of the patient in order to combat cancer, that weakness gives reign to the cancer to spread. He advised walking in fresh air and teaching patients how to breathe in the air.[68] He felt that the physician should have the attitude of defeating the cancer, that he (or she) needed to hold a fixed idea that he would be victorious over the disease. Jones also believed that after careful evaluation of the patient and his or her condition, a treatment plan should be adopted that is right for that patient. Then, both physician and patient should stick to that plan.

He cautioned against anything that would lower the vitality of the patient. All medicines must work in harmony with Nature or they will lessen the chance of recovery. Nature is the ally in the treatment and must be invoked. Excessive amounts, even of good medicine, assault vitality. Careful observation of the patient on a daily basis is the only way to be certain that the cure is working as desired. He spoke words that are all too familiar nearly a hundred years later: "Many doctors treat disease as an enemy that must be expelled from the system by force of arms. No remedy is too powerful for them. They speak of their heroic treatment, of the big doses of medicine, and tell of the wonderful cures they have made."[69] He felt these claims were spurious and that a valid treatment has to concern itself with the disease, the medicine, and the vitality of the patient.

In very difficult cases, Jones also advised practitioners to hold a few good remedies in reserve, ones that could be called into service after the first treatments had run their course.

The Jones Escharotic Method

At the time Jones was writing, many practitioners used escharotic pastes for the treatment of cancer. Jones believed that escharotics constituted local treatments whereas the remedies and adjunctive treatments, such as the diet and epsom salt baths, were systemic. Jones firmly believed that it is impossible to cure cancer using a local treatment such as an escharotic. He stated emphatically that the growth is merely the local manifestation of a constitutional disease.[70] As such, removal of a tumor involves removal of the effect rather than the cause. As Jones developed more experience in the treatment of cancer, he came to depend less and less on the escharotics and more on the systemic treatments.

Jones also opposed the practice of cutting away a portion of the tumor after use of escharotics because he believed that any kind of cutting irritates the tumor and makes it grow faster. For the record, my understanding of this is that Jones regarded cancer as a sleeping lion one did not wish to awaken. If the portion that is cut is dead, as with the Fell and Pattison techniques, this would not seem to fall under the Jones admonition to avoid the knife. Most

likely, the more modern Mohs Method is also an exception since only dead tissue is removed. However, it should be emphasized that Jones himself did not combine any form of surgery with his escharotics, but he often used considerably more paste than others whose work has reached my attention.

The formulas for the escharotic pastes used by Jones as well as his poultice powder, healing salve, and figwort syrup are given in appendix B. It will be noted that several of his escharotics are more chemical than botanical.

Though there are many nuances in the usage of the various Jones escharotic pastes, the normal method was to use a paste for about two days on a smaller tumor or five to six days on a larger one. Jones said that there is more danger in discontinuing the escharotic too soon than in leaving it on too long. It is important that the paste reaches deep enough to necrotize the entire tumor. For the most part, the paste will not act on healthy tissue. If there is glandular swelling, *phytolacca* (poke root) poultices should be used to reduce the swelling. In any event, the mass itself is poulticed until the eschar detaches. Sometimes this was followed by applications of phytolacca cerate. Then, if the area seemed clean and free of morbid matter and malignancy, the yellow healing salve was applied. Jones maintained that the area would not close and heal if cancer were left in the treatment site—or, if the area did heal, it would break open again. He always urged against premature efforts to close a treatment site, writing in one instance, "It is just as impossible to heal up a cancer sore as it would be to heal a volcano."[71]

He stated that anyone can remove the tumor; however, *skill is required to adapt the local treatment to the changes in appearance that occur from day to day*. Occasionally, he required five months of treatment before declaring the patient permanently cured.

BREAST CANCER

Jones treated more cases (4300 cases) of breast cancer than any other type of cancer. This was, as we recall, also the situation for Pattison and Fell as well as many others. Historically, the escharotic method was one of the preferred treatments for breast cancer. The largest tumor Jones ever removed was a breast mass measuring twenty-two inches in circumference and weighing four and a half pounds.

FIBROID TUMORS

Jones claimed to be the first physician in the U.S. to treat fibroid tumors by medicinal means. He found that this condition is best resolved by *phytolacca.* For the indigestion accompanying it, he used *hydrastis* (goldenseal); and for hemorrhaging, he used *aqua cinnamon.* He made a mixture of two parts fluid extract of phytolacca, one part fluid extract of hydrastis, one part bicarbonate of soda, and a pint of aqua cinnamon. He administered a teaspoonful three times a day before meals. He felt that lime checked the growth of the tumor by changing the condition of the blood. The treatment may need to be continued for six months to a year.

In other cases, Jones gave a tincture of *fraxinus* (ash), ten drops three times a day, and iodide of lime, one-third grain once every three hours for a week, then two-thirds grain every three hours. For pressure on the bladder that obstructed the flow of urine, he gave *Solidago virga aurea* 1X, five drops every three hours.

PHYTOLACCA DECANDRA

Some of the Eclectic physicians used *Phytolacca decandra* (poke root) as an escharotic. Jones considered it to be the most valuable remedy available for the treatment of cancer.[72] He sometimes used a "soft extract" (or solid) of fresh green poke root, sometimes mixed with equal parts of solid extract of *Sanguinaria canadensis* (bloodroot) and red clover flowers. When he used this escharotic instead of one of the others, the procedure was essentially the same: the escharotic was applied until the malignant mass was destroyed. The area was then poulticed until the eschar detached. If the area was clean and free of signs of malignancy, it was healed with the yellow salve.

Jones also used juice of sheep's sorrel and birch leaves. In general, these remedies did not go deep enough to destroy the whole tumor. Moreover, they are quite painful. He wrote that he tried acetic acid, alcohol, solution of zinc chloride, caustic potash, double chloride of gold and sodium, chromic acid, and many other remedies that he injected into or near the tumor—but all these he put aside for treatments he regarded as superior.

Jones warned that care should be taken when exposing the bone through escharotic use. Nature, he said, can only cover a small surface of exposed bone. If too much is exposed, skin grafting will be necessary.[73]

SAFETY

On page 145 of his book, Jones described a case of a tumor on the neck directly over the jugular vein. He treated this in essentially the same fashion as other masses, without risk to the vein.

PAIN

With some of the escharotic pastes and certain applications of the paste, pain is a major factor. Jones sometimes added opium powder to the escharotic to reduce pain.[74]

REMEDIES

Jones used a variety of remedies for very specific conditions. He gives the indications for use of each remedy in chapter 10 of his book. Throughout his book, he describes the actual treatments used with various patients. His usages are summarized below.

ACETIC ACID

For cancer of the stomach. "Dissolves cancer cells in the stomach."

APOCYNUM CANNABINUM (American hemp)

Growths in the breasts where there are small bunches that are movable and hard like "a rubber ball." Quarter ounce of apocynum to one ounce of lanolin. Mix and rub into the breast three times a day.

ARNICA MONTANA (leopard's bane)

For breasts that are sore after bruising or injury. One part arnica to three parts glycerine. Rub into the breasts three times a day. INTERNALLY: use homeopathic Arnica montana

BAPTISIA TINCTORIA (wild indigo)

For last stages of cancer when there is prostration. Also for fetid discharges. DOSE: five drops every two hours.

BELLIS PERENNIS (English daisy)

Breast tumors when the growth has been caused by injury and the tumor is of recent origin. DOSE: ten drops, three times per day.

BORO EUCALYPTOL

Apply three times a day to scar tissue when recurrence in cicatrix appears.

BRYONIA ALBA (European white bryony)

For breasts that are heavy and hard and where motion increases the pain. Alternate with phytolacca. DOSE: five drops of tincture with six ounces of water. One teaspoonful an hour. CAUTION: *this herb is poisonous. Do not exceed recommended dosage.*

CANCER DROPS

Phytolacca, thuja, and baptisia in equal parts. DOSE: ten drops every three hours.

CELASTRUS SCANDENS (staff vine or climbing bittersweet) ointment
A vanishing ointment for tumors of the breast. One pound of green leaves to two pounds of lard and one ounce of beeswax. Simmer over a hot fire for a few moments. Rub into the breast day and night.

CHELIDONIUM (greater celandine) tincture
For liver cancer when the urine has a strong odor. DOSE: five to ten drops, three times a day.

CHIMAPHILA UMBELLATA (pipsissewa)
For women with large breasts, retracted nipple, pain in the tumor, and glandular involvement. DOSE: ten drops, three or four times a day, gradually increasing the dosage to twenty drops. After one month, change to tincture of goldenseal, thuja, and poke root: ten drops every three hours. For bladder cancer where there is bloody pus and mucus in the urine, give ten drops every three hours. See also eucalyptus.

CINCHONA (Peruvian bark)
Jones mentioned this remedy but did not explain his use of it. The bark is sometimes known as Jesuit's powder and has traditionally been used as a febrifuge. It is high in alkaloids and quinines.

COLLINSONIA (stone root)
For fullness and pressure in the rectum. Mixed with water. DOSE: one teaspoonful every hour.

COLOCYNTH (*citrullus colocynthis*) tincture
This is a highly poisonous substance that can cause death. Jones put ten drops in a six ounce glass of water (or five drops in a four ounce glass of water) and gave a teaspoonful of the mixed fluid every hour or two to patients with stomach cancer (near pyloric valve) or pancreatic cancer attended by severe shooting pains extending into the bowels. *Not to be continued for more than one or two days.*

CONDURANGO TINCTURE
For breast cancer patients who have ulcers in the corner of the mouth or painful cramping in the stomach. DOSE: five drops every three hours.

CONSTIPATION #1 [75]
Podophyllin, $1/4$ grain; aloin, $1/5$ grain; extract of nux vomica, $1/8$ grain; extract of colocynth, $1/8$ grain; oil of capsicum, $1/8$. DOSE: one pill at bedtime.

CONSTIPATION #2
Aloin, five parts; extract of belladonna, five parts; podophyllin, two parts; and ferri sulphate, eleven parts. DOSE: one pill at bedtime.

CONSTIPATION #3
Podophyllin, five grain; leptandrin, twenty drains; hydrastin thirty grains; nux vomica, five grains. DOSE: one pill at bedtime.

CORYDALIS FORMOSA TINCTURE (turkey corn)
For advanced cancers where the lymphatic glands are swollen and the face has dry, scaly scabs. DOSE: ten drops four times a day. Also for cachexia. DOSE: ten drops of the tincture, three times a day.

DIOSCOREA TINCTURE
For stomach cancer with gas and griping pain. DOSE: sixty drops in a wineglassful of hot water. Repeat in an hour if needed.

Echinacea (purple cornflower)

For the pain of liver cancer and in the last stages of other cancers to ease the pain. Mix half ounce echinacea tincture with six ounces of water. Dose: teaspoonful every hour.

Eclectic wash

Fluid extract of baptisia and fluid extract of lobelia herb, zinc sulphate, and water. One teaspoon in a cup of warm water, apply to gauze, and press against tumorous mass. Use one teaspoonful to a pint of water as douche or enema with cancer of the lower intestine. Retain as long as possible (30-60 minutes) and increase strength of the mixture with successive uses. Can also be used with abscesses.

Epsom salts

Used in baths and as compress on breast tumors where there are lumps in the axilla.

Equisetum hyemali tincture

Bladder cancer. Urinary distress with severe pain after voiding, extreme and frequent urination. Dose: fifteen drops every two hours.

Eucalyptus globulus cerate

Extract of eucalyptus mixed with equal amount of salicylic acid. Mix with vaseline and apply as a compress to large breast masses where there is pain but no ulceration. Change dressing three times per day. Where there is ulceration, use cerate of eucalyptus and iodoform. Spread on a soft white cloth and apply over the diseased surface three times a day. It will stop the smell and later the sore will have a healthier appearance.

Eucalyptus globulus tincture

For stomach cancer with vomiting of blood and sour fluid, give twenty drops morning and night. For desperate cases of bladder cancer, give twenty drops of the tincture every three hours. See also *Chimaphila umbellata*.

Galium aparine (cleavers, wild bedstraw)

Cancer of the tongue when there is a lump in the tongue or nodular feeling to the tongue which is tender and painful, especially at night. Dose: twenty drops of tincture every three hours or four times a day. Also use a mouthwash of the tincture, diluted one half with water once every two hours. Retain in the mouth for several minutes. Can be painted directly onto the tumor. May need to be continued for several months.

Gaultheria hispidula (cancer wintergreen)

In cachexia, capable of eradicating the diathesis towards cancer. One ounce of the herb to one pint boiling water. Half a wineglass three times a day. Tincture can be made by adding one pound of fresh herb to one pint 80% alcohol. Let it stand one week and filter. Dose: one teaspoonful, four times a day.

Geranium maculatum tincture

For hemorrhaging associated with stomach cancer. Dose: $1/8$ ounce every hour until the bleeding stops.

Germicide

This is used as an antiseptic for the stomach and bowels and to destroy germs. It is given in advanced stages of the disease where the tongue is coated. It is made of four parts dolomite lime, one part magnesium sulphate, and half part sugar and administered in tablet form. DOSE: one tablet an hour for eight hours, then one tablet in three hours or one after each meal and at bedtime.

GOLDENSEAL (*Hydrastis canadensis*):
For cancer of the stomach where there is distress after meals, flatulence, and the tongue is coated with yellow slime. DOSE: ten to twenty drops every four hours. Can be alternated with Acetic acid in homeopathic potency (1X five drops every four hours) and acetic acid compress to exterior of abdomen.

GOLDENSEAL-BAPTISIA-THUJA
For breast cancer with bloody discharges from the nipple. DOSE: ten drops every three hours or twelve drops after each meal.

GOLDENSEAL-HEMLOCK
Used on large breast tumors that have spread to the axilla. Four parts solid extract hydrastis to one part solid extract conium. Spread on thin white leather and apply directly to breast. Change plaster every forty-eight hours. This treatment reduces the mass so that the use of an escharotic is possible. Jones followed this treatment with his paste no. 1.

GOLDENSEAL-PHYTOLACCA
Equal parts of the tincture for hard tumors of the breast. DOSE: ten drops after each meal.

HYOSCYAMUS (henbane)
For nerves. Small doses in lieu of opiates. *This is poisonous.*

IODO BROMIDE CALCIUM
For large cancers of the breast. Mixed with three parts water, applied to cloth, and placed on the breast.

IRIS VERSICOLOR TINCTURE (blue flag)
Tumors of the uterus. This tincture was used for enlargement of the spleen as well as exophthalmic goiter. Take fresh roots, mash them, and add eight ounces to a pint of 80% alcohol. Let the mixture stand for fourteen days, then filter. DOSE: twenty-five drops three times a day.

JAMAICA DOGWOOD
Pain due to large uterine growths. DOSE: thirty drops every four or eight hours depending on the pain.

LIVER PILLS
Podophyllin, five grains; leptandrin, twenty grains; extract of nux vomica, five grains; extract of gentian (as much as necessary). Used to overcome constipation. DOSE: one at bedtime.

NITRIC ACID
For painful swellings of the submaxillary glands.

NYMPHAEA ODORATA (white pond lily)
Cancer of the uterus. Mix with phytolacca and *Helonias dioica* root. Make a gallon of syrup. Give a wineglassful three times a day. As a remedy for the blood, Jones was of the opinion that it could not be excelled. Note: Maude Grieve mentions poultices and douches of this herb for uterine cancer as well as boils, tumors, and other afflictions of the skin.

Phytolacca folium cerate (poke)

Ulcerated cancer near the eye with discharge. Spread on a soft white cloth and apply three times a day. The cerate should consist of approximately 20 percent juice of poke leaves mixed with vaseline.

Phytolacca cerates

For recurrences in the scar tissue of breast cancers. The treatment may require three months. For breast cancers where the lump is hard and knotty, use cerate of equal parts of the juices of phytolacca, arnica, and belladonna. Rub into the breast at night and spread some on white cloth and apply after rubbing. This ointment is absorbent. Can be combined with homeopathic Calcarea flouride, 6X. Also, take one teaspoonful of tincture of goldenseal, hemlock, and poke root every three hours. Continue the internal treatment for two months after disappearance of the mass.

Phytolacca poultice

Equal parts poke root, slippery elm, and lobelia seed. (In some instances, Jones omitted the slippery elm or used only phytolacca. In other cases, he used baptisia instead of lobelia seeds. In yet other cases, he used only slippery elm and lobelia seeds or only slippery elm and flax seeds.) Change every three to twelve hours or moisten with fluid extract of phytolacca and lobelia seed and change every other day. (Jones sometimes used only phytolacca tincture to moisten the poultice.) The treatment often needs to be continued for three to five months.

Phytolacca lotion

Use equal parts phytolacca root and glycerine. Rub into enlarged tonsils three times a day.

Phytolacca syrup

Fluid extract of two parts green root of phytolacca, and one part each of gentian extract and dandelion extract. Jones said it supported the appetite and strength, especially in older patients. Used for breast cancer where the breast is hard "like old cheese." It can also be used for tumors of the throat, uterus, and rectum. He also administered this syrup to patients with tongue cancer but added five grains of potassium iodide to each dose of the syrup for these patients. Dose: one teaspoonful after each meal.

Phytolacca tincture

Used primarily in breast cancer when the breast is hard and painful and of a purplish hue. Dose: five drops of the tincture every three hours. Can be alternated with Kali muriaticum 3X, three tablets every three hours. Can also be added to poultice powders when there is hard swelling. Mixed with iodine, it can be painted externally on exophthalmic goiter.

Phytolacca-helonias dioica (false unicorn) tincture

For uterine-cervix cancer. Helonias is a blood maker. Dose: ten drops every three hours.

Phytolaccin-sanguinarin pill

Pill made of $1/8$ grain sanguinarin and $1/4$ grain phytolacca. This is used for cancer of the rectum where there is looseness of the bowels, anemia, and low vitality. In some cases, Jones used only phytolaccin. DOSE: one pill every three hours. If the mouth becomes dry, reduce the dosage. Jones sometimes used *jatropa* (bull nettle root) in these tablets, $1^{1}/_{2}$ grains jatropa to $^{1}/_{4}$ grain phytolaccin.

SANGUINARIN

For cancer of the rectum. DOSE: one-eighth grain every three hours.

SANGUINARIA (bloodroot) NITRATE

For cancer of the tongue where there is ulceration on the side. One grain nitrate sanguinaria to one drachm of glycerine. Pour out two to three drops of this mixture on a glass plate. Take a glass rod and dip it in the drops on the plate and apply to the ulcer after first having cleaned it with cotton. Be sure the area is clean before treating. Treat three times a day.

SCROPHULARIA MARYLANDICA (figwort)

Valuable in advanced stages of cancer when there are lumps in the neck and axilla. See the Compound Syrup Scrophularia in appendix B.

SEMPERVIVUM TECTORUM (houseleek)

One part tincture to eight parts glycerine. Use as mouthwash, once every two hours for tongue cancer where the side of the tongue is painful and ulcerated. Press cotton dipped in the wash against the growth and hold in place for a few minutes, three times a day. It is important to be persistent. In a stronger solution, one part sempervivum to two parts glycerine, it can be painted directly on the affected parts three times a day.

SLIPPERY ELM POULTICE

For uterine-cervix cancer. Put the slippery elm in a porous bag, press directly against the cervix after the malignancy has sloughed off. Change every twelve hours.

SPIGELIA

For burning and unbearable pain associated with cancer of the sigmoid. Fifteen drops of tincture of spigelia in half a glass of water. Give one teaspoonful every half hour. (For lancinating pain, see colocynth.)

STILLINGIA SYLVATICA (queen's delight):

For bronchial irritation. Four parts stillingia to sixteen parts wild cherry syrup. DOSE: one teaspoon every two hours.

STRAMONIUM DATURA (thorn apple) OINTMENT

One and half pounds of leaves to two pounds of lard. Boil gently for an hour. While still hot, strain through coarse linen and add two ounces of melted beeswax. Stir until cool. Use on indurations around open sores; also for lumps in the breast. Rub in well twice a day.

SUPPOSITORY #1

Cyripedin, two parts; *scuttellarin*, two parts; extract of *hyoscyamus*, one part; butter cacao. One suppository in the rectum day and night. For cancer attached to bowel as well as cancer of the rectum. Can also be used to relieve pain at night. One suppository before bed.

SUPPOSITORY #2

Iodoform, five parts; extract of eucalyptus, two parts; extract of hamamelis (witch hazel), two parts; cocoa butter. For ulcerations of the rectum with indurations. Insert one per night.

Use in conjunction with the Eclectic wash (as an enema) three times per day.

Thuja tincture

Jones injected ten to twenty drops of this tincture directly into tumors of the vagina, cervix, and rectum, every other day, until the tumor sloughed off. This procedure was followed by painting a mixture of thuja and glycerine (equal parts) directly onto the diseased surface, three times a day, until the sore healed or inserting a tampon of thuja tincture into the vagina and changing it twice a day. Internally, the patient was given a tincture of thuja or thuja and phytolacca, ten drops every three hours. This treatment may cause elevation of temperature and increase in pulse rate. Jones gave thuja tincture, four parts to six parts water, to patients with bladder cancer. Dose: one teaspoonful every three hours.

Thuja salve

One part oil of thuja to ten parts vaseline. Apply directly to ulcerated areas of rectum.

Thuja-Conium-Hydrastis-Phytolacca tincture

Equal parts. Fifteen drops before each meal. Given to patients with cancer attached to bowel.

Ustilago maidis

For certain fibroid tumors in the early stages of growth when hemorrhage is a prominent symptom and when the blood is dark with many clots. Dose: ten drops, three times a day.

Veratrum veride (green hellebore)

This is a poisonous plant. Indications: hard pulse. Very small doses. Note: Maude Grieve states that the dose is one to three minims every two to three hours. A minim is one-sixtieth of a drachm which is an eighth of an ounce. In other words, the amount used is infinitesimal. Jones recommended this remedy for the early stages of congestive lung cancer: five drops in four ounces of water, a teaspoonful an hour. The frequency of administration is reduced at the slightest signs of nausea. This remedy can also be administered in homeopathic 1X dilution, ten drops every hour for three hours, then once every three hours until the pulse feels soft and regular.

Viburnum (guelder rose) Compound

For stomach gas. Dose: one teaspoonful in half a cup of hot, sweetened water, every fifteen minutes as needed.

White pinus canadensis

For throat cancer. Two parts each: extract of white pinus canadensis, borax, and glycerine to eight parts water. Gargle every two hours or spray the throat using an atomizer.

Homeopathic Remedies

NOTE: *Jones described the protocols used on a wide range of patients. I listed these and then compared them to his own descriptions of the remedies used in his treatments. In certain instances, there were discrepancies in potencies and dosage and occasionally even in the indications. The reader is advised to consult a competent homeopath to determine if and when any of the remedies mentioned here are suitable in his or her particular situation.*

ACETIC ACID 1X

Cancer of the stomach or bowels. DOSE: five drops every four hours along with constant compress of the same to the external surface of the stomach.

APIS MELLIFICA 3X

Used when there is pain of a burning or stinging nature and in breast cancer where there is induration and the skin is dark purple and discharges are light yellow. DOSE: twenty drops to half a glass of water. One teaspoonful every hour.

ARNICA MONTANA 3X

For trauma. DOSE: ten drops every three hours.

ARSENIC IODIDE 3X

For breast tumors when the breast is indurated, painful, and sensitive to the touch, especially if the tumor has begun to ulcerate. Used when the axillary glands are swollen and hard or when there is an exudation that forms a brown crust. Also used for epithelioma of the lip.

ARSENICUM KALI 3X

For cauliflower excrescences of the uterus with smelly discharges, pressure below the pubis, and pain.

ASTERIAS RUBENS 3X

For fleshy persons of lymphatic temperament with breast cancer attended by lancinating pain. Indications: flabby with red face; breasts that are swollen and distended before the period; and/or a very red spot appears on the breast that is ulcerated and has foul smelling discharges. DOSE: five to ten drops every three hours.

AURUM 6X

Cancer of the nose with greenish pus or discharges. DOSE: three tablets, four times a day.

AURUM MURIATICUM NARONATUM 3X

For fibroid tumors of the uterus when there is a discharge of yellow mucus from the vagina, decreased flow of urine, loss of appetite, melancholy, and burning pains in the abdomen. DOSE: three grains one hour after each meal.

BARYTA IODIDE 3X

Used where the growth is hard but not ulcerated; with adenoid (movable, hard lumps) forms of cancer; and with breast cancer of longer growth. DOSE: three tablets every three hours. Can be alternated with ten drops of Hydrastis 3X. Also for ovarian tumors with a scrofulous taint to the system (no mention of alternating with Hydrastis) and for enlarged, hard goiter.

Belladonna 1X

Used for breast cancers when the pain is worse from lying down. Dose: five drops every three hours.

Bismuth 2X

For cancer of the stomach attended by vomiting of clear fluids or when enormous quantities of food are ejected from the stomach that seem to have stayed in the stomach for days. Can also be used when there is burning and pain in the stomach. Dose: three tablets every two hours.

Bromine 6X

Use when the lymphatic glands under the jaw are hard. Dose: five drops every three hours.

Calcarea carbonica 3X

For persons with cancer who have a tendency towards boils, cold feet, and copious putrid, white discharges, who catch colds easily and whose hands and feet perspire. Dose: three tablets every three hours.

Calcarea Flouride 6X

For those with breast cancer where the tumor has been long standing and is hard and knotty. Jones also administered this remedy to some patients with stomach cancer. Dose: three tablets every three hours.

Calcarea iodide 1X

For cancer of the breast when the growth is tender; when there are sharp, darting pains; and when use of the arm on the affected side increases the pain. Dose: three tablets every three hours. For uterine fibroids, give $^1/_3$ grain every three hours.

Carbo vegetabilis 3X

For cancer of the stomach where there is flatulence and the stomach feels full and tense from gas that causes more pain when lying down. Dose: three tablets every two hours.

Causticum 2X

For cancer of the stomach when the flesh is very tender over the abdomen and the patient cannot even bear clothing to touch the area and when even the lightest food or pressure cause violent lancinating pain. Dose: five drops every two hours.

Chelone glabra 1X

Indigestion. Dose: three tablets every three hours.

Chinum arsenicum 3X

For watery, painless diarrhea; emaciation; and burning in the rectum associated with cancer in the intestines. Dose: three tablets every two hours.

Cholesterinum 3X

For liver cancer where the liver is enlarged and there is burning pain on the side, sallow complexion, emaciation, yellow conjunctiva, and the patient holds his or her hand on the side while walking. Dose: six grains once every four hours, three tablets every three hours, or six grains three times a day.

Condurango 2X

For cancer of the stomach accompanied by cracking at the corners of the mouth and severe, cramping pain in the stomach, especially at night. Dose: five drops every three hours.

Conium maculatum 2X

Breast cancer where the breast is stony hard, where there are stabbing pains, and where the breast swells up during menstruation. It does not check growth but this remedy eases pain. DOSE: ten drops every three hours or five drops every two hours.

Ferrum 1X

For anemia, emaciation, and blood loss. DOSE: three tablets every four hours, sometimes alternated with *thuja tincture*.

Ferrum picrate 3X

After prolonged use of alteratives, use to build up iron in the blood. DOSE: three tablets after each meal and at bedtime.

Graphites 3X

For conditions of the nose where there is a tendency towards ulceration. DOSE: three tablets every three hours.

Hecla lava 6X

For hard, bony tumors of the jaw. DOSE: three tablets four times a day.

Hydrastis canadensis 1X (glycerine based)

For lupus with ulceration of the skin. Apply to the skin every three hours. Take ten drops internally every three hours. Also on breasts when there is dyspepsia, constipation, and/or flatulence. DOSE: ten drops every two hours. (See next entry.)

Hydrastis canadensis 3X

For cancer of the breast with lancinating pain and indigestion, dyspepsia, constipation, and flatulence. DOSE: five to ten drops every three hours or ten drops after each meal.

Hydrocotyle asiatica 1X

For what Jones called lupus, a kind of cancer of the skin in which there is significant change in the structure of the skin without ulceration. Use where there is profuse perspiration and thickening of the skin attended by exfoliation of scales and dry eruptions. DOSE: five or ten drops every three hours. Can also use with cancer drops. Add one part tincture to three parts glycerine and paint over the diseased surface three times a day. (Compare to *Hydrastis canadensis 1X*.)

Iodine 6X

For cancer of the stomach when there is rapid emaciation, hunger that is not relieved by eating, and the patient feels worse in a warm room. Also used for cancer of the pancreas and for exophthalmic goiter. DOSE: ten drops in a little water once every two hours.

Iodoform 3X

Cancer of the left lobe of the liver. May be alternated with Cholesterinum 3X, one dose of each, every four hours (i.e. a dose of one or the other every two hours.)

Kali bichromate 3X

Ulcers of the septum that are painful to the touch accompanied by secretions that are tenacious and stringy as well as loss of appetite and when the condition is worse in cold weather. DOSE: three grains every three hours.

Kali cyanatum 3X

In last stages of cancer of the tongue when the pain is severe and very little nourishment can be taken. DOSE: one grain, three times a day.

Kali Muriaticum 3X or 6X

Used when there is white fur on the tongue and bunches in the breast of recent origin that feel soft and tender. Can also be used for constipation. Dose: ten tablets at bedtime or three tablets every three hours.

Kali phosphate 3X

Use after the tumor has been removed and the skin is "tight as a drum" during the healing process. Dose: three tablets every three hours. Can be alternated with Silicea 6X, same dosage.

Kali sulphate 3X

For small epithelioma on the face with scabs; a red, angry appearance; and watery yellow discharges. Dose: three tablets every three hours along with a salve of equal parts Kali sulphate and vaseline. Use three time a day.

Kreosotum 3X or 6X

In uterine cancer when there is burning in the pelvis and a discharge of foul smelling blood clots. Dose: three tablets after each meal and at bedtime. (See next listing.)

Kreosotum 6X

For stomach cancer attended by vomiting of sour, dark-colored fluids after eating and when there is burning pain. Dose: three tablets after each meal and at bedtime.

Lachesis 6X

Cancer of the breast where the growth has a purplish appearance, is open and fungoid, and when the breast bleeds easily and the blood is dark and decomposed. Also for use with uterine-cervix cancer when there is hemorrhaging and loss of dark, decomposed blood; and for ovarian cancer when the pain extends from left to right and is relieved by blood flow from the vagina. Dose: dilute ten drops in half a glass of water and give one teaspoonful of this mixture every hour.

Lapis albus 6X

For fibroid tumors with intense burning pains and profuse hemorrhaging or malignant uterine tumors with black bloody discharge. Dose: three to five tablets every two to three hours or three times a day. Also indicated when there is enlargement of the lymphatic glands but they feel soft and are movable.

Murex purpura 6X

Cancer of the uterus attended by acrid discharges, swelling in the thighs, pain that feels as though it were created by a sharp instrument, and depression. Dose: ten drops, three times a day.

Muriatic acid 3X

For advanced cancer of the tongue. Dose: fifteen drops in half a glass of water, a teaspoonful every two hours. Relieve pain with Kali cyanatum 3X, two tablets night and morning.

Nitric acid 3X

For rectal pain where there is a feeling of burning pains or tearing after elimination. Also for pain and swelling of the submaxillary glands. Dose: fifteen drops to half a glass of water, one teaspoonful every two to three hours.

Nuphar lutea 2X

For morning diarrhea associated with cancer of the intestines. Dose: five drops every two hours.

Nux vomica 2X or 6X

For vomiting of sour fluid from stomach. Also for indigestion associated with fibroid growths. Dose: three tablets every three hours.

Phosphorus 6X

For hemorrhagic diathesis, slight wounds that bleed easily. Dose: fifteen drops to half a glass of water, one teaspoonful every two hours.

Picrotoxine 3X

Night sweats associated with cancer of the intestines. Dose: two grains at 5:00, 7:00, and 9:00 p.m.

Sempervivum tectorum 2X

For ulcers of the mouth or tongue that are characterized by soreness, stabbing pain, and bleeding. Dose: five drops in a little water every three hours. Also, use dilute solution (two parts water to one part remedy) and apply locally.

Sepia 6X

For burning, throbbing pain associated with uterine-cervix cancer. Also for cancer of the lip that bleeds easily. Dose: three tablets every three hours alternated with phytolacca-helonias tincture.

Silicea 6X

In "superficial" cancer or cancer of the glands where there is a thick, yellow offensive discharge. Also for breast cancer where the nipple is retracted and there are fistulous ulcers of the breast. Dose: three tablets, three or four times a day.

Solidago virga aurea 1X

For obstruction of the flow of urine due to pressure of tumors. Dose: ten drops every four hours.

Staphysagria 3X

For ulcers and tumors of the nose where the limbs also feel bruised. Dose: ten drops every three hours.

Terebinthina 3X

For tenesmus, burning pain, and hemorrhage associated with bladder cancer. Dose: five drops every two hours.

Thuja 30X

Used to remove the poisoning of the blood caused by vaccination that Jones said exhibited as eruptions on the face, swelling in the axilla, and lumps in the breast. Dose: three grains a day or three tablets three times a day. Also used for cauliflower cancers of the uterus, fungous growths, cancer of the throat (equal to phytolacca in importance) and tumors of the rectum. Jones often injected thuja directly into the tumor or the surrounding tissue.

Ustilago 1X

For cervical tumors that are soft and spongy and bleed easily when touched. Dose: three tablets every three hours.

CHAPTER 9

Understanding Choices

*E*ARLIER EDITIONS OF THIS BOOK did not contain instructions for using the salves. Patients and practitioners insisted not only that the book have instructions but that the instructions stem from my own judgments based on the years I have spent investigating escharotic treatments of cancer. I do not actually regard myself as an expert, certainly not in the sense that Pattison, Jones, Nichols, or Mohs were experts. However, unlike these clinically grounded physicians, I have an overview that entitles me to some hypotheses, even if the assumptions or presumptions are both qualified and preliminary.

We recall that Pattison was first influenced by Justamond and Girouard who used arsenic based compounds. Then, he used the "hybrid" formula—bloodroot and zinc chloride—that he later came to reject in favor of a much calmer goldenseal preparation. Fell and Pattison initially used equal parts of bloodroot, zinc chloride, flour, and water. Even if we allow for the fact that the water and zinc chloride have such an affinity for each other that they quickly

blend into one compound (not necessarily a saturated solution), it should be recognized that these pastes were milder than the ones typically marketed today. The proportions in Hoxsey's famous red salve are not known, but the Mohs fixative paste is about one-third zinc chloride. Jones used a variety of pastes. The mildest had one part each of zinc chloride and chromium chloride to twelve parts bloodroot and one part glycerine. The strongest, used on breast cancer, was a saturated solution of zinc chloride and carbolic acid that was added to another paste that contained twelve parts zinc chloride to seven parts other ingredients.

This is quite a range, and I believe it is appropriate to recognize that using the same paste for everyone is just a little bit too simplistic. Though most producers do not divulge the exact ingredients much less the proportion of each in their "black salves," most readily available pastes are fifty percent zinc chloride. In my opinion, these pastes are far too aggressive for lay use. Moreover, they are hugely painful and unpredictable.

Bloodroot is a very interesting and precious herb, but it is unlike almost anything else of a botanical nature in that it is so quickly absorbed into the blood stream. It therefore becomes a systemic treatment the moment it is used. Personally, and I realize this is highly controversial, I would prefer to see bloodroot used in very moderate dosages internally—and only *very* rarely used in external preparations

This is a big statement and one likely to provoke a lot of backlash from producers of black salves and Compound X formulas as well as satisfied patients. However, in taking this position, I feel that I have merely retraced the experience of Pattison and come to similar conclusions.

Bloodroot is so unpredictable and inflammatory that there is no way to estimate its potential action once applied to the skin. This said, it may do nothing at all. There may be no reaction whatsoever, but it may become so systemic that excruciating pain and fever are almost immediate—and anything in between these two extremes is also possible.

No one wants pain, but fever can be good for patients if the fever is high enough. Inflammation, however, is not, *in my opinion*, desirable. I agree with Pattison that it may increase blood supply to the tumor—so that between the irritation and additional nutrients, the tumor may become more active.

Since launching my Web site, hundreds of people have written me about their experiences with bloodroot pastes. Several claimed to be cured; some were not certain. A few resorted to surgery when they realized the tumor was growing faster than the methods they were using to destroy the tumor were working. One woman was severely disfigured, a consequence that could surely have been avoided had she been better informed, had she used some other product, and had her methods been completely different.

In contrast to bloodroot, goldenseal is elegant and precise. Several professional herbalists doubt my findings. They recite pages and pages of studies attesting to the anti-cancer properties of bloodroot—and challenge me to cite similar studies in favor of goldenseal. The debate is however purely academic since only clinical comparisons will reveal which herbs to use under which circumstances.

In the meantime, I remind my colleagues that bloodroot and goldenseal were both once called *puccoon*. The use of red puccoon was learned from Native Americans in the Lake Superior area; and the use of yellow puccoon stemmed from contacts with the Cherokee peoples. Writers often did not differentiate the particular puccoon to which they were referring, but Pattison was unmistakable: he used the botanical names of *Sanguinaria canadensis* and *Hydrastis canadensis*. He treated thousands of patients with bloodroot before changing to goldenseal—and he modified the technique, not a little, but a lot. Though his enucleating paste contained twenty-five percent zinc chloride, he diluted the paste with nine parts calendula ointment. The amount of zinc chloride in the first application was thus truly modest.

Only as the nerves became numbed did he increase the potency of his preparation.

Those who have stayed with the material in this book are, of course, by now aware that there are many techniques for using escharotic products. These vary from (1) single application methods without bandaging, to (2) a dual strategy involving the alternation of escharotic and drawing salves, to (3) methods as complex and sophisticated as those of Pattison, Jones, Nichols, and Mohs.

Simply stated, with my present understanding, I believe that, *in lay hands*, the use of a single salve, such as a Compound X formula, is only appropriate for relatively small basal cell carcinomas. In professional hands, the issues may be slightly different, but it should be remembered that the physicians who used such pastes believed that years of experience were required before these products could be used correctly. Moreover, we can even divide these experts into two schools. On the one side, we place physicians such as Nichols and Mohs who used highly aggressive products swiftly. This is only possible when there is a capacity for pain management. Nichols did not divulge his formula, but I suspect it was purely chemical, not botanical at all. On the other end of the spectrum, we have Pattison—and probably Hildegard of Bingen. Jones was somewhere in between.

When using an aggressive product, it is important to act decisively so as to minimize stimulation of the tumor. In favor of such strategies, it must be admitted that if the tumor is fast growing, it may be necessary to move quickly—though, this said, I fear there is still a possibility of aggravating the tumor so that it grows faster than it is necrotized.

Throughout most of this book, I have suggested that the strength and painfulness of the escharotic depends mainly on the amount of zinc chloride in the formula. However, this is not strictly true. Both zinc chloride and bloodroot are escharotics in their own right. Native Americans used bloodroot and roasted red onions to destroy tumors—and the method was painful even without zinc chloride.

Goldenseal does not hurt and is not an escharotic. It is very quiet in comparison to bloodroot. It does not promote inflammation; moreover, many who use it report that their tumors were significantly reduced (and closer to the surface) after only one day of use. On the downside, goldenseal is slow, very slow compared to bloodroot. I had trouble adding up all the days in each stage of Pattison's treatment, but he mentioned that some patients stayed in his rooms for five months. I have no doubt at all about this, but those who use the method of alternating the black and yellow salves also often spend five to seven months with treatment, all the while risking that irritation is aggravating the growth of the tumor, risking that scar tissue will form making contact with the remaining tumor difficult, and suffering all the while with pain and uncertainty.

It is difficult to know how well Pattison's method works on very simple conditions, such

123 *Understanding Choices*

as basal cell carcinomas. Experts mainly used escharotics on breast tumors, and Pattison was no exception. It is also impossible to know how well Pattison's method works if scratches are not made in the eschar. Most patients are too squeamish to make these little scratches, but if this step is omitted, it is not clear that the paste will penetrate deeply enough to necrotize the entire tumor in one round of treatment. When the eschar does fall off, a residual is almost certain to be there if the scratches were not made. The Pattison method is therefore a professional technique rather than a lay procedure.

OBJECTIVES

In order to present essentially sound instructions, a few more preliminary statements are required. First, the escharotic technique is really an alternative to surgery. It has objectives that are comparable if not identical to surgery: an effort is made to remove the malignancy with minimal damage to surrounding tissue. In fact, the salve has been used to amputate gangrenous structures—as well as to avert surgical amputation by healing the diseased areas. Yes, it has traditionally been used with both such ends in mind.

Second, there are many stages to the process. More subtle methods employ different products during each of the stages.

Third, people and tumors are different. One woman writing over the Web described three lesions on her body. Two were successfully removed with a black salve she herself made, but the third did not react to the salve.

Blind loyalty to a single product is simplistic and foolish.

Fourth, given the enormous range of products used over the centuries and throughout the world, there is, in fact, scope for modifications of both products and techniques. Therefore what I will present is merely one adaptation, and a flexible one at that. Moreover, I will assume that the tumor in question is a breast tumor though the same strategies can be used with most other malignancies.

Knowing that I am not exactly on *terra firma*, I wish to make the premises of these directions clear. As I said, compared to most others, I have somewhat of an overview. I have researched the history of escharotic treatments, understand many of the reasons for the diversity of techniques and products, and thus feel qualified to a few opinions. However, this said, I am quick to go on record stating that I am not a medical doctor and that most of my ideas are "composites" or purely theoretical. On the other hand, they address the most serious deterrents to use of this method.

I will present a goldenseal method because I personally regard it as superior to the bloodroot methods. Though the procedure is obviously based on Pattison, it is another "hybrid" approach, perhaps aged and matured by the passage of almost one and a half centuries.

Pattison maintained that goldenseal has a specific effect on cancer that is deeply constitutional. My assessment is that goldenseal arrests the fermentation surrounding the tumor and thereby deprives the cancerous mass of the nutrients upon which it depends for survival.

Conceivably, and this is pure speculation, it also inhibits circulation to the tumor as it is much more contracting than inflammatory. I suspect that these factors "buy time" in such a way as to justify the use of a softer technique that takes longer.

This said, my experience is that this method cannot be used after aborting use of the bloodroot pastes. Many have shared with me their frustrations with bloodroot products. Once the tumor has been irritated, it is necessary to be resolute, either with a more skillful bloodroot technique or surgery. In most instances, goldenseal will not penetrate fast enough to the bottom of the tumor where growth is occurring (see page 57). At least three people who contacted me after using bloodroot wound up having surgery. One was a medical doctor who even with the pain relieving products available to her was not able to use the paste aggressively enough.

PREPARATION

Since escharotic and enucleating methods need to be continued, there are some preliminary measures that might be tried. Where tumors are not growing rapidly, it is worth considering internal protocols before embarking upon the external. Hildegard recommended a minimum of three days of yarrow tea. Pattison and Jones relied heavily on their internal remedies, so much so that ninety percent of those they saw in the latter years of their careers were cured by these methods

alone. There are similar reports from the Biomedical Center in Tijuana, the clinic that carries on the work of Harry Hoxsey. These measures obviously take time, months, but they are certainly worth considering.

Secondly, it is wise to make a dummy bandage with something comparable in texture to a salve to see how use of a dressing for several months might affect movement and morale. I have suggested that people use the worst possible dressing, turmeric and flax oil. This is very challenging as the oil loosens the bandage and the turmeric stains—and constitutes a crash course in reality.

Many have sent me e-mail saying that they are absolutely committed to using salves to treat their cancers, that they are not quitters, and that they have reasonable tolerance for pain. I usually suggest that they try a poke ointment similar to those described by Jones before making up their minds. Several wrote back saying the pain was unbearable, this when no skin was blistered, no wound was created that might have to remain open for months, and no zinc chloride was used!

I am not trying to dissuade anyone from using escharotics, I am merely trying to set out the facts before the point of no return is reached. Also, I am not inferring to anyone that their desire to pursue a more natural path of treatment is flawed, nor that they are unable to take more charge of their own healing. I am merely helping people to realize what they are getting into before it becomes difficult to extricate themselves from their choices.

CHAPTER 10

Instructions

THE DIRECTIONS THAT FOLLOW are for an enucleating technique. There is scope for varying the approach depending on the size and depth of the tumor, product preferences, and speed that the mass is growing. As a general rule, this method is not recommended for tumors that are fast growing nor for those that have metastasized. Though supervision and/or monitoring is advisable, it is not readily available. *Anyone employing these methods does so at his or her own risk.*

PRELIMINARIES

Regardless of the type of cancer, extent or stage of its growth, and method of treatment, most of those who used escharotics—from Hildegard of Bingen, Native American medicine men and women, to Harry Hoxsey—suggested that patients take suitable internal tonics. The exceptions to this rule were those, like Perry Nichols, M.D., who denied that the disease is systemic in nature and who therefore relied exclusively on their escharotic treat-

ments. Though physicians as a whole tended to see cancer as a localized condition, among those who used botanical salves, most viewed cancer as a systemic disease. Hildegard recommended a yarrow beverage as both a preparation for use of her violet salve and as a preventative against metastasis, the dread of all patients. She also suggested a duckweed elixir and *anguillan*, a quite elaborate internal tonic that she said caused the "viruses" in the body to get sick and die.

Native Americans subscribed to a similar doctrine and protocol: correct the patient's digestion and eliminate the poisons that stem from poor digestion, purify the blood, and support deep inner healing. The historic Eclectic formula, *trifolium compound*, was no doubt learned from Native Americans as was the currently popular Essiac preparation. Interestingly, burdock was an ingredient in all these tonics, but not in the *compound syrup scrophularia* of Dr. Eli G. Jones. Though most such tonics were prepared as elixirs, i.e. they were sweetened, some were taken as teas.

Some of the tonics have more anticancer properties than others; all aid digestion, lymphatic movement, and elimination. Hoxsey recommended that his tonic be continued for life, but the dosage was reduced when all systems of the body were normalized. Since so many attributed their high cure rates more to the internal remedies than the escharotics, wise patients will listen!

EXTERNAL APPLICATIONS

Some patients may also want to try some less drastic external treatments before committing to an escharotic or enucleating course of action. These preparations vary considerably and correct use depends upon the condition. Some are intended for use on ulcerated lesions, some on lumps that are deep. Some are more useful where there is congestion, others where there is infection.

Hildegard's violet salve was used on everything from muscle soreness to ulcerated tumors. Native Americans often decocted herbs and used these as compresses. There was a formula from Virginia, published in 1734, that utilized sassafras and dogwood. Pipsissewa was another of the herbs used in this way. Christopher made a fomentation of mullein and lobelia. I have sometimes suggested that people use *coptis*, a Chinese herb with some properties similar to goldenseal. It reduces inflammation quite quickly.

Some practitioners employed poultices. The more aggressive of these used fresh green poke root, sometimes mixed with other herbs, such as bayberry, baptisia, lobelia, or red clover. Tinctures were also used as topical applications or to moisten poultices that were becoming too dry to be effective. Dr. William Fox made a liniment of blue flag, red clover, and bloodroot. This is applied to clean linen or gauze and changed as necessary, sometimes every two hours, sometimes only after twenty-four hours. The poultice must be kept moist.

Finally, there are ointments and/or oils that can be applied topically. Again, many of these contain poke root, but there is a wide range of choices here as well. In a significant number of cases, these methods will be sufficient to remove all evidence of cancer; however, there are situations in which these methods will not be adequate and something more will be required.

What is important to note is that while escharotic treatment is an alternative to surgery, these other remedies can generally be used in addition to surgery should someone prefer this option to others. Moreover, a few of these herbs promote proper healing of surgical incisions. Jones had an ointment that he used on recurrences in scar tissue.

CANCEROUS CONDITIONS

In the twelfth century, Hildegard and her mystic brothers of the cloth in Tibet described miniature organisms that cause cancer. To-date, there is no conclusive proof of a viral link to cancer, but it is accepted that approximately eighty percent of the cancerous mass is not malignant. The rest of the mass consists of infection and other morbid material. Those who used escharotics described profuse discharges of purulent matter. If the nature of a tumor were better known, it is clear that more specific products could be developed. In the meantime, most with experience in the matter believe that the external preparations change the terrain sufficiently to deprive tumors of what they need for growth. In other words, a salve might be a combination of something that relieves infection, arrests fermentation and the anaerobic processes upon which the tumors depend for nutrients, and something that actually attacks and destroys the tumors more directly. The salve may also contain something to relieve pain.

Designing the Salve

Goldenseal is probably the premier antimicrobial herb in North America. As early as 1798, Benjamin Smith Barton reported that the Cherokee were curing cancer with the roots of this marvelous plant. Scientific studies indicate that goldenseal destroys cancer mainly by increasing macrophage activity.

Turmeric is another multipurpose herb. It inhibits the tendency of cells to divide, reduces almost all the odor associated with cancer, and significantly relieves scarring. It can be taken internally as well as externally. It is however somewhat tricky to use because it lacks the mucilaginous characteristics of goldenseal.

With these two herbs as primaries, the rest of the formula can be devised according to need. If pain is the primary concern, white willow bark can be used. If angiogenesis is the major issue, burdock might be tried. If there is a suspicion of parasitic involvement, black walnut is an option. Some people want to use violet leaves or flowers, red clover blossoms, and/or poke root in the basic salve. Others have added everything in the basic Essaic formula or just sheep's sorrel. Some use white oak bark.

There is no precise right or wrong here, but it is important to find what works and no two people are precisely the same. A simple salve with powdered goldenseal root (5 parts), turmeric (4 parts), and white willow bark (3 parts) with calendula oil works just fine.

The herbs need to be blended. Some people, following suit with Fell and Pattison, use flour. Others use only the powdered herbs and oil or water. I use oil because of its superior capacity to penetrate.

I make several different kinds of oils. I start with cold pressed apricot kernel oil because of the potential benefit of the nitrilosides. I then add herbs to the oil. For pain relief, I make an oil with white willow bark. For spasm, I use marigold flowers. For its anti-infective properties, lomatium can be tried. Use just enough oil to make a thick mixture. I also add a special ingredient, a calendula paste made with a carbon dioxide process.

The salves then need a small amount of curing. I suggest using a yoghurt maker because the temperature stays constant around 98-105°F. Put the salve into the jars for twenty-four hours. They are then ready to use. Though they do not need refrigeration, this may be good when hot weather makes the salves runny.

This simple salve often shrinks tumors quite quickly; it does not, however, blister the skin. To turn the salve into an enucleating ointment, zinc chloride is used. Though everyone else mixed the zinc chloride into the paste, I prefer to put a teaspoon of zinc chloride into an empty one-ounce eyedropper bottle to which distilled water is added. It is then very easy to adjust the potency of the basic salve to the needs of the individual by using anywhere from a few drops to considerably more depending on sensitivity, the stage of the treatment, depth of the tumor beneath the surface of the skin, and reactivity of the tumor to the salve. *Do not touch any metal object to the zinc chloride.*

This salve is quiet by the standards of everyone else's products. It is not aggressive, but it is capable of doing the job, albeit slowly. It should *not* therefore be used with tumors that appear to be growing fast.

To Make the Salve

- Goldenseal powder
- Turmeric powder
- White willow bark (or *di da wan*)
- Calendula oil or ointment or other oil (white willow bark or lomatium)
- To add to the escharotic
  - calendula CO_2
  - homeopathic *Apis mellifica* or *Arnica montana*
- Yoghurt maker
- Glass containers

Preparation

- Yarrow tea for three or more days before starting.

While Waiting

If you have not already done so, now is a good time to experiment with the dummy dressing and bandaging. The first issue is choosing where to apply the salve. There may be choices.

In the illustration below, it can be seen that by applying the salve closer to the nipple, the distance to the tumor is shortened. However, it is possible to go from somewhat higher and avoid some of the risk of removing part of the areola or nipple. It may lengthen the treatment time by a few days but make bandaging easier while also serving the patient's desire to remain more in tact.

While waiting for the salves to cure, it is important to gather the rest of the items needed to proceed.

WITH A MASS DEEP INSIDE BREAST, THERE MAY BE CHOICES OF WHERE TO APPLY THE PASTE OR SALVE. IF THE NIPPLE IS NOT INVOLVED AND PRESERVATION OF IT IS A CONCERN, APPLYING THE SALVE HIGHER WILL AVOID RISK TO THE NIPPLE BUT PERHAPS PROLONG REACTION TIME.

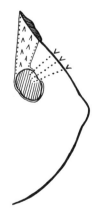

For first stage

- •Enucleating salve
- •Zinc chloride
- •Wooden applicator
- •Hydrogen peroxide, colloidal silver, or witch hazel
- •Sterile cotton balls and/or gauze
- •Occlusive bandage
(large enough to cover the application site with overlap of at least one inch on all sides)
    - •Conventional bandage
    - •Plastic wrap of some type
    - •Cloth impregnated with beeswax
    - •White leather
- •Tape (paper or waterproof)
- •Pain relievers (optional)
    - •To use orally
    - •To use directly on site
    - •Homeopathic *Arnica montana* and/or *Apis mellifica*

ADVICE

• Do not engage in any vigorous activity or lift heavy objects using the side of the body being treated.

• Avoid increasing circulation such as may occur by taking extremely hot baths or going out in the hot sun.

Not being an expert on homeopathic remedies, I am hesitant to make suggestions. However, since the initial treatment is bruising, homeopathic *Arnica montana* may be considered. Later, most escharotics are more burning. *Apis mellifica* might provide some relief at this stage. Homeopathic remedies can be added to the escharotics and/or taken orally. For further information, read the list of homeopathic remedies used by Dr. Eli G. Jones (pages 116-120) or consult a qualified homeopathic practitioner.

OCCLUSIVE
Air tight, closed bandage.

FIRST STEP

It is important to decide exactly where the paste will be applied. Take into account:

- •Where the tumor is
- •Whether the entire mass can be covered with the paste
- •Gravity
- •Whether there are choices in application sites
- •How far beneath the skin the mass is
- •How the area can be bandaged
- •How bandaging will affect movement
- •Whether, with movement, the bandage will remain air tight or leak
- •Whether the application site is near a nerve plexus or gland

Starting

Check to see that everything that will be required is available. Review the instructions and warnings to be certain this is a treatment you wish to pursue. Then, prepare the salve.

•If adding a pain reliever and/or homeopathic remedy to the paste, mix them in before applying the paste.

•The paste should be thicker than toothpaste but malleable. If too thin, the paste can be thickened with turmeric powder —which, however is crumbly. If too thick, add more oil or pure water.

•Clean the treatment site with hydrogen peroxide, colloidal silver, or witch hazel.

•Apply a thick layer of the escharotic paste with a wooden applicator.

•Cover the site with the occlusive bandage. Be sure to have at least an inch of tape surrounding the salve.

•Leave the bandage in place for twenty-four hours.

Comments

If possible, the entire mass should be covered. To minimize the risk of growth of the primary tumor and/or metastasis, it is also advisable to avoid an increase in circulation to the affected area. Use of milder products, less zinc chloride, will make this more feasible.

Since the treatment will probably take several months, it is important to consider how bandaging will affect movement. If uncertain, do a harmless trial with a dummy application (see page 125). Try to take into account how close the treatment site is to a nerve plexus since proximity to nerves is likely to increase the need for serious pain management. If the treatment site is near lymph nodes or glands, it may be even more important to keep inflammation to a minimum.

Patience

1. Wait twenty-four hours before removing the bandage.

2. If the site becomes very painful, take pain relievers.

3. If there is a systemic reaction, drink a detoxifying tea and be certain to support proper elimination.

4. Reduce stress as much as possible.

5. Rest, especially if a fever ensues.

Response to Initial Application

It is almost impossible to estimate what sort of reaction will occur with the first application—or for that matter any subsequent application. Be prepared to experience anything from mild tingling or prickling sensations to itching or burning or rather acute pain. Some people run systemic fevers and a few have nausea. Much depends on the preparation used and the patient's individual response to using that particular product.

DRESSING CHANGES

- Hydrogen peroxide or witch hazel or colloidal silver

- Cotton balls, swabs, or gauze

- Hygienic disposal method

- Occlusive bandages

After approximately twenty-four hours, carefully remove the bandage and whatever salve is still on the treatment site. Be gentle since the area will be sensitive.

- Avoid any jostling or rough treatment!

- Clean the site with hydrogen peroxide, colloidal silver, or witch hazel

If the water supply is clean, bathing after removing the dressing and before applying a fresh dressing to the site is all right; however, do not direct forceful streams of water to the site, and do not rub the site. Do not use soap on the eschar (it is fine to use soap to remove adhesives from the skin surrounding the eschar.)

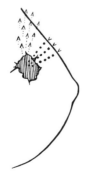

THE ESCHAROTIC MUST PENE-TRATE THROUGH THE HEALTHY TISSUE UNTIL IT REACHES THE TUMOR. THEN IT MUST DESTROY THE ENTIRE TUMOR.

WHAT TO EXPECT

If the treatment area reacted with the escharotic, there should be anything from tiny blisters—pinhead size to small bubbles—to solid areas that are whitish, yellowish, green-ish, or greenish-gray. If no reaction appears on the surface or if there are only a few small dots that have formed, continue as previously:

1. Prepare another application of enucleating salve, this time adding twice as much zinc chloride as the first time. Apply this to the site with a wooden applicator.

2. Cover with an occlusive bandage.

3. Have pain relievers on hand.

4. Wait an additional twenty-four hours.

5. Remove the dressing after twenty-four hours.

6. Clean the treatment site with hydrogen peroxide, witch hazel, or colloidal silver.

7. Examine the site to determine the degree of the reaction.

8. If the entire area has not blistered, repeat the entire process (for a third time). The amount of zinc chloride used in the application should be gradually increased until an eschar starts to form.

After the Blistering Appears

If the growth is small and on or near the surface of the skin, a single application of an escharotic is sometimes enough. If the lump is bigger, it is important to persevere until the entire lump is necrotized. Moreover, once starting the treatment, it should be continued since irritation of the site may stimulate the growth of whatever part of the mass remains in the treatment site. *Do not abort the process.*

As the process advances, the blisters on surface area will form into a more solid eschar that gradually becomes harder and thicker and usually also darker. At a certain point, further salve applications will probably rest on the surface of the eschar without penetrating through the thickened, dead tissue.

At this juncture, it is essential to determine how far the escharotic has penetrated and whether in all likelihood the entire tumor has been destroyed. If only the most accessible part of the tumor has been necrotized, it may be necessary to make scratches in the eschar in order to force the salve to penetrate the dead eschar and reach the tumor under the eschar. Failure to do this may necessitate additional use of the escharotic in the open area after the eschar has detached.

Basically, no product is capable of penetrating a thick eschar, even if oil is added to the preparation. Therefore, the choices are basically simple: (1) make the scratches in the eschar (which is completely painless); or (2) wait for the eschar to detach, but be prepared for several rounds of treatment.

Many patients believe that the eschar, the first eschar, they see is the tumor. However, in all likelihood, it is mainly surface skin with perhaps a little necrotized tumor. This is especially true if the tumor is deep.

Making the Scratches

As previously noted, many people do not want to make scratches. What people need to understand is that the eschar consists of dead tissue. However, it may be quite thin or rather thick. If cuts are made in a thin eschar, there is, of course, risk of bleeding. Though the salve will stop the bleeding quickly, irritation of the living tumor should be carefully avoided. Using a very sharp scalpel and magnifying glass will allow for precision in this somewhat delicate task.

Nevertheless, if confidence is lacking, this procedure is best left to experts—in which case, an eschar will form and detach and expose residual tumor. This is not a crisis, merely the consequence of the choice not to make any scratches or cuts. If one uses an escharotic instead of enucleating product, the same probability of having residual malignancy exists.

Formation of the Eschar

With either method, the eschar will continue forming. The issue is simply what to do while this is happening. Use of more enucleating salve will be useless unless it is penetrating the eschar. Therefore, unless the scratches are made, it is likely that there will be a few days when nothing is happening on the surface and no serious use of products is required—though, in my opinion, the area should be covered with some ointment and protected from infection. For this purpose, a violet or calendula ointment can be considered. Herbal compresses or poultices are additional possibilities. These can be used in such a way as to overlap the treatment area with fairly wide margins; this will not increase the size of the eschar.

Since experts do not agree on which method is superior, one must simply choose a product and a strategy and follow through with the decision. This said, it is my belief that someone who starts with this somewhat modified Pattison technique, and who then decides either that the process is dragging on too long or that a more aggressive method is preferable, may switch to a Jones technique—and product. However, the reverse is not true. If one begins with a highly inflammatory paste, one must use a method that is suitable to such a product and seek quicker results.

CRACKING AROUND THE EDGES

During the next stage, the eschar will show signs of separating from the surrounding tissue. This usually begins with a well-defined perimeter that eventually becomes a crack whose width and depth continue to increase until the eschar finally detaches.

The "crack" is sensitive, but initially, at least, it is seldom open even though oils and ointments penetrate well through this tissue.

Once the crack becomes a real crack rather than a line, discharges may occur. These can be anything from simple serous fluids that are thin and watery in appearance to thick purulent matter that may consist of necrotic tissue, liquefied tumor, and/or infectious matter.

Pattison felt that these fluids promote separation so he tended to avoid applying dressings at this stage. I feel that it is necessary to keep the area active and sterile. Therefore, I developed a product for use in the cracks. I named it *Golden Myrrical* because it is made with goldenseal, myrrh, and calendula.

The process for making this product is similar to that of making the salves, but I use castor oil and Irish moss instead of apricot kernel oil and turmeric. This salve works very well for at least five days. It prevents closure of open sites, promotes liquefication and discharge, and protects against infection. Several health care professionals have begun using it on very deep tumors, such as occur in the breast and the liver or pancreas. It seems to delay separation of the eschar but promote healthier separation of the tumor from the supporting tissue.

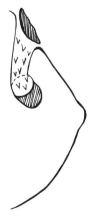

THIS DRAWING SHOWS AN ESCHAR FORMING ON THE SURFACE OF THE SKIN AFTER HAVING NECROTIZED THE TOP OF THE TUMOR, BUT THE GREATER PART OF THE TUMOR IS STILL UNAFFECTED BY THE TREATMENT.

The Crack

Pattison and Jones used a variety of dressings once the crack began to open. In my estimation, it is extremely important to keep the area clean and disinfected. The choice of an ointment or poultice depends mainly on the amount of discharge. Poultices[P] are used to "mop up" purulent matter. Basically, there are wide choices as to which herbal products to use. Some patients describe severe itchiness, usually worst around the time of the full moon. Others have more heat than itching. A few just feel an increasing sense of weight. This latter is due to the death of the tumor. It feels heavier as it begins to separate.

This is a stage of treatment with many nuances. Pattison described the little cuts and how he put fairly concentrated enucleating paste both into the cuts and the cracks. He also described use of a calendula ointment that overlapped the eschar and surrounding tissue. Between these two stages, he apparently did nothing. Jones, on the other hand used only an escharotic until the eschar detached.

All this is quite understandable unless approaching this method for the first time. Since the Jones method goes fast (and uses a significant quantity of escharotic paste), the eschar detaches in a few days. However, with the Pattison technique and products, the eschar may take a month or more to detach. In the meantime, the crack keeps widening. If the tumor is large, there will come a time when one can see the edge of the tumor as well as the surrounding tissue and observe how the separation is occurring. This is, of course, nothing short of fascinating. By using *Golden Myrrical* at this time, the crack becomes a major source of discharge and cleaner separation is probable. It is difficult to say how often to use this product. In general, it promotes profuse discharge after the first few applications; then, reactions to its use decline. When discharge is heavy, a poultice can be used for a day or two and then the *Golden Myrrical* can be used. If the process slows down, more enucleating salve can be inserted into the crack. Usually, it can be applied with a wooden instrument or small paint brush though some prefer to use strips of clean linen. This keeps the process active when necrotization and discharge seem to be slowing down.

Unlike lay use of the bloodroot salves, when using this method, the eschar tends to be thick—and thus the crack can also be quite deep. It surrounds the tumor; and, as the ointment moves downwards between the tumor and supporting tissue, it promotes proper separation or *enucleation*. When the process takes a long time, it can be assumed that the tumor is large and deep.

For the record, under no circumstances should the yellow healing salve be used for more than a day or two until the treatment site is ready to be closed. This salve does tug at the eschar; and, to this extent, it aids separation, but it also promotes healing. This should not be permitted unless the eschar has detached and there is nearly total certainty that the

---

[P] See appendix B for poultice formula used by Dr. Eli G. Jones. Add turmeric to the poultice to keep scarring to a minimum.

entire tumor has been removed. Anything else causes premature closure, excessive scarring, and the trapping of residual in the treatment area. It is thus almost guaranteed to result in what is normally called a recurrence. It is not, of course, a recurrence; it is merely an incomplete treatment. It will be recalled that Fell reported a recurrence rate of about thirty percent using his method. Pattison had a recurrence rate of approximately fifteen percent. It is difficult to compare these figures with surgicial recurrence rates since types of cancer, the stage at the time of treatment, and measurement intervals play important parts in interpreting the statistics. Pattison's figures are nevertheless impressive and perhaps superior to modern statistics on breast cancer recurrence.

DETACHMENT OF THE ESCHAR

The event that everyone eagerly awaits is the detachment of the eschar. It must be permitted to fall off on its own without any prompting. With a small growth, separation may occur after only a few days, but a large breast lump will probably take several weeks. If the tumor is very large, pieces may fall off before the entire eschar separates. Sometimes, the eschar seems to be hanging on by a mere thread. It must not be pulled off before it is ready to detach on its own.

As soon as the eschar falls off, the site underneath will be clearly visible. It will be bloodless and usually remarkably clean and pinkish. Sometimes, the newly exposed area

appears to be flat, as if it regenerated before allowing the eschar to detach. Other times, there is a significant crater. Often, but not always, there is a hole at the bottom of the crater from which morbid material is discharged. This material is usually greenish-gray in color and has a decidedly unpleasant odor. It is important that the hole remain open so long as the discharge continues. Poulticing at this juncture serves several purposes: it keeps the area clean, draws out morbid material, and prevents the site from closing. Jones often used poke root poultices at this stage. This is aggressive and almost as painful as a bloodroot paste. He also used a gentler poultice made of equal parts of slippery elm bark, lobelia or baptisia seeds, bayberry root bark, and flax seeds. Pattison continued with his use of goldenseal, as a diluted enucleating paste, powder, or infusion (see page 95). He, too, often used poke root. When the discharge subsides, my *Golden Myrrical* can be used. This salve is absolutely painless. Alternating various preparations is possible at this time, but only good judgment will minimize the chances of recurrence.

SITE INSPECTION

Perhaps the single most important part of the entire escharotic process is the proper observation of the crater after detachment of the eschar. Sometimes very tiny greenish-gray patches can be seen with the naked eye or with the help of a good magnifying glass. Sometimes, there are several such small spots and sometimes there are larger suspicious areas.

If any tumor remains, the enucleating salve must be reapplied. Once the tumor is accessible, as after the eschar detaches, the salve does not have to be used full strength. However, it needs to make direct contact with the remaining malignancy. It can be painted on these spots or "packed" into the crater, depending on how much appears to be remaining. Unless the salve is quite diluted, it will hurt. However, the modified Pattison salve is usually well tolerated—even at this stage, it causes less pain than a toothache.

INTERPRETING THE RESIDUAL

The fact that there is some tumor remaining in the treatment area does not imply that the method failed nor that the technique was inadequate. It can happen whenever the tumor is large or deep, when too little of the enucleating salve was used, or when scratches in the eschar were not made properly or this step was omitted. No matter what the explanation, it is crucial that these residuals are necrotized while there is easy access to them.

If there are only a few tiny spots, the escharotic can be applied directly to those spots (being careful to apply the preparation to a larger area than the visible tumor.) The rest of the crater can be filled with a calendula-goldenseal mixture (without zinc chloride) or *Golden Myrrical*. The site should be bandaged. A second eschar will form, usually smaller than the original one. It will also usually detach faster. While waiting for it to form, the procedures are essentially the same as the first time.

The enucleating salve should be used until the tumor is necrotized. Poultices are indicated when there is discharge, and *Golden Myrrical* can be applied to assist separation. The area should be kept occlusive, and dressings should be changed at least every day. If there is profuse discharge, poultices sometimes have to be changed every two to four hours.

This cycle is repeated so long as there is evidence or suspicion of remaining malignancy. When completely satisfied that destruction of the entire tumor has occurred, healing can be permitted. At this time, the treatment site should be free of discharges and odor, and it should appear entirely clean and pinkish. To be extra certain, it may still be wise to apply poultices or ointments for a few more days. At this stage, many people enjoy Hildegard's salve. It has a pleasant aroma and clean feeling. Some like to use Christopher's black ointment, *German Kermesberro*, since it has poke root, but is not as intense as the fresh green root or tincture. Others use fomentations or liniments of anticancer and/or detoxifying herbs. Some use *termentina*, an ointment made of pine pitch. There is no right or wrong at this point. Patients are usually both exhausted by what they have been through as well as relieved. Most are busy "reclaiming their lives" because they see life after cancer. Many are more conscientious at this stage than earlier because they realize they have futures to create.

My personal view is simply that even after reasonable doubt has been eliminated that several days be devoted to meticulous cleansing of the treatment area.

CLOSING THE TREATMENT SITE

After a long process, the time to close the area arrives. This is remarkably easy. It sometimes occurs in a day or two. However, to minimize scarring, turmeric should be added to the healing ointment. Most people like to add aromatic oils as well.

Pattison used various derivatives of pine pitches. Jones had a yellow healing salve (see appendix B). Christopher had his black ointment. Lay persons have a yellow healing or drawing salve. I make several different salves, all pleasant. For a day or two, these should be applied thickly and held in place by an occlusive bandage. Later, they can be gently rubbed into the treatment area and surrounding tissue.

AVOIDING RECURRENCE

No one can promise that cancer will never return. There are simply some measures that reduce the likelihood of a second bout with cancer. In my estimation, these involve attention to stress, diet, metabolism, elimination, and any changes in the treatment site.

Hoxsey supplied his internal tonic for life: patients were to continue taking it as long as they lived. Early in his career, he made this available for a one-time fee, but this is no longer the situation. It makes sense to me that people with a history of cancer commit either to such life-long use or to periodic detoxification and tonification twice a year. It also makes sense that general health measures are implemented that reduce risk.

I would also advise patients to observe the lymphatic glands in the areas surrounding their treatment, making sure that the glands are not engorged or tender. Lymph tonics and teas, fasting, and adhering to a diet of foods that are readily digested will ease the burden on the lymphatic system.

Applying occasional fomentations to the old treatment site is also a way of paying respect to a part of the body that was once very sick and wounded. Occasional use of such plasters or ointments makes a lot of sense to me.

FOLLOW UP

Finally, there is a need to determine how well the treatment went. Approximately two to four months after treatment, it would be appropriate to have some non-invasive tests of the blood and perhaps also the treatment area. These can include the AMAS test or another blood test specific to the type of cancer treated—or a dark field microscope analysis of the blood. Ultrasound can also sometimes be highly reliable.

Since new developments in technology are always occuring, I will try to keep information on how best to follow up as well as on the availability of herbal products posted on my Web site.[q]

---

[q] See http://www.cancersalves.com for up-to-date information.

Site inspection is the way to assess the success of the treatment with salves (or pastes). This step is ignored by nearly all lay practitioners and providers of escharotic pastes; however, it is the judgment upon which life may depend. Just as a surgeon may or may not remove the entire malignancy, it is possible to remove a piece of a tumor and leave the rest, including the roots, in place. Since irritation of the mass may aggravate growth, no part of the tumor should be allowed to remain in the treatment site. The assumption that a single round of salve use will result in death of the entire tumor is naïve. If there is any evidence at all of remaining malignancy, the entire process should be repeated until the area is completely clear. As a general rule, it is better to use too much of the salve rather than too little and to continue longer rather than to abandon the process.

THE ORIGINAL SUSPICIOUS GROWTH WAS ABOUT THE SIZE OF A THUMB NAIL. THE BLACK PASTE WAS APPLIED SO AS TO COVER THE LESION COMPLETELY AND OVERLAP THE EDGES BY ABOUT HALF AN INCH (ONE CENTIMETER MORE OR LESS). NOTE HOW THE OCCLUSIVE BANDAGE IS APPLIED (TEGADERM™) — THE STIFF PAPER IS REMOVED (SEE NEXT PHOTOGRAPH.)

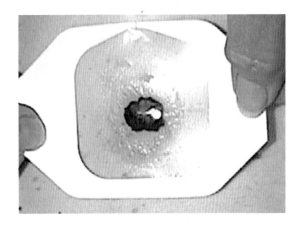

NOTE THAT THE PASTE IS APPLIED THICKLY AND THE COVERING OVERLAPS THE PASTE BY A CONSIDERABLE MARGIN. THIS PREVENTS LEAKAGE AND SPREADING. SEE THE TOP WHERE THE BANDAGE ENDS. THE PASTE IS LEFT IN PLACE FOR 24 HOURS.

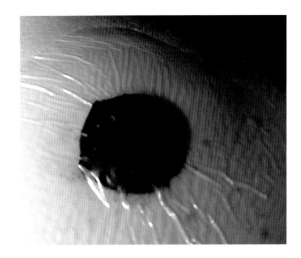

REMOVAL OF THE PASTE AFTER 24 HOURS. NOTE THAT THERE HAS NOT BEEN A REACTION ON THE FIRST PART EXPOSED AFTER APPLICATION (THE PASTE OVERLAPPED THE SUSPICIOUS LESION BY A CONSIDERABLE MARGIN.) THERE IS MODERATE INFLAMMATION AND REDDENING. THERE WAS A SMALL REACTION WITH THE ACTUAL LESION (NOT SHOWN ON THIS PICTURE.)

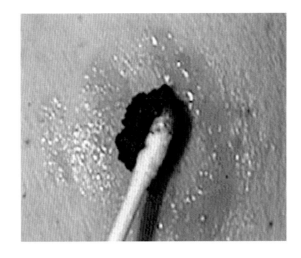

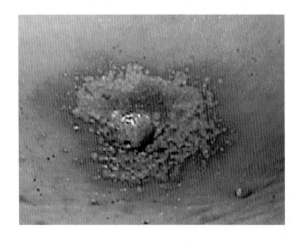

TYPICAL REACTION TO USE OF AN ESCHAROTIC PASTE. NOTE THAT WHERE THE REACTION WAS MINOR, THERE ARE TINY BLISTERS WHEREAS THE SUSPECT AREA (AND JUST ABOVE IT) WAS MORE REACTIVE TO THE SAME PASTE. A REACTION SUCH AS THIS MAY OCCUR IN AS LITTLE AS A FEW HOURS TO AS LONG AS FOUR TO FIVE DAYS. THIS ONE TOOK TWO DAYS.

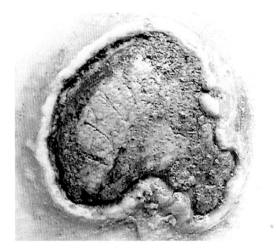

DAY 13, NOTE THE TINY SCRATCHES IN THE ESCHAR. SINCE THE ESCHAR IS COMPLETELY DEAD, MAKING THE SCRATCHES CAUSES NO PAIN WHATSOEVER. WITH EACH DAY, IT IS POSSIBLE TO MAKE DEEPER AND DEEPER CUTS.

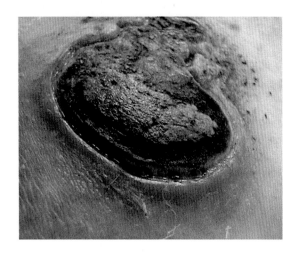

DAY 11. THE ESCHAR HAS REACHED ITS MAXIMUM REACTIVE DIMENSIONS. IT IS THICKENING. THE EDGE IS BECOMING MORE DEFINED. THERE CONTINUES TO BE SOME INFLAMMATION AROUND THE PERIMETER, EXTENDING FOR A SMALL DISTANCE. THE ESCHAR ITSELF IS DEAD, BUT IT IS STILL VERY MUCH CONNECTED TO THE SURROUNDING TISSUE.

Filling the crack around the edge. Approximately Day 11. The preparation contained goldenseal, turmeric, and calendula oil. It has a consistency similar to mustard.

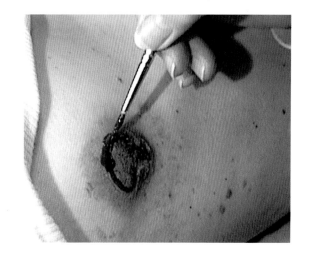

Recurrence in scar tissue after surgery for breast cancer that included removal of many lymph nodes. An enucleating salve was used in a wide area. The reaction occurred along the scar tissue. This picture clearly shows the cracking and separation of the eschar from the supporting tissue.

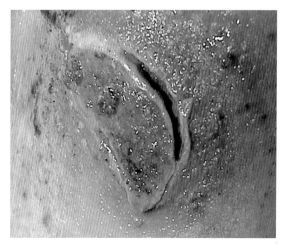

The treatment site immediately after detachment of the eschar. Same patient as above. Note that the site is absolutely bloodless, clean, and relatively flat—as is typical with enucleating salves. Despite the healthy appearance, there was profuse purulent discharge for many weeks.

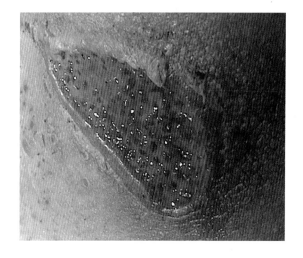

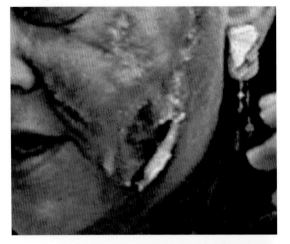

Partially detached eschar. This is a case of inoperable angiocentric T-cell lymphoma (the tumor was wrapped around the artery.) One technique for working with such tumors is to work along a line, opening one part and then the next and next. The escharotic, a black salve in this case, did no harm at all to the artery.

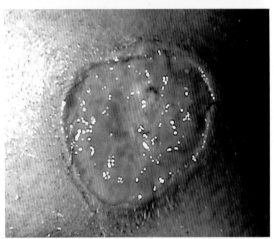

Example of purulent discharges. These discharges are sometimes profuse. In general, they indicate the need for profound detoxification and immune boosting as well as external use of poultices containing anti-infective herbs.

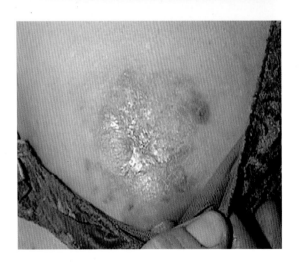

Healing of the treatment site. At this stage, the escharotic/enucleating process is complete. However, it is advisable that anti-scarring ointments be used, that poultices be applied occasionally to the entire treatment area so as to maintain tissue health in the original tumor site and surrounding area, and that internal tonics be used for at least two to five years, if not for life. This patient had a lump somewhat larger than a walnut that she had ignored for many years.

This picture illustrates the use of the salve as a post-surgical treatment. The patient had breast implants (see surgery line on the left) and two lumpectomies (surgery scar in the middle below the eschar that is forming.) An enucleating salve (without zinc chloride) was used on the entire breast (which was severely inflamed.) The reactive area was limited to either side of the lumpectomy scars. Residual malignancy was confirmed via ultrasound tests.

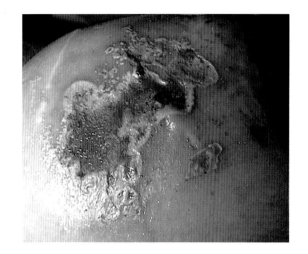

This is the treatment site after detachment of the eschar (different photographic angle.) The lumpectomy scar tissue shows as a line through the middle of the eschar. Note how remarkably clean the treatment site is. It is also extremely flat, a condition that is typical with enucleation.

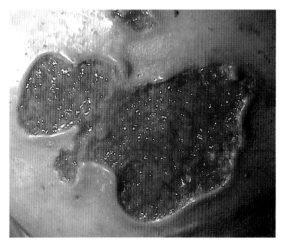

The site after the second round of enucleation. Though the tumor was reactive to the salves, the need to remove the implants dictated surgery. The patient elected to deal with both the implants and malignancy surgically in order to speed up the resolution of her condition. Despite her decision, post-surgical use of a mild enucleating salve is something many persons may wish to consider.

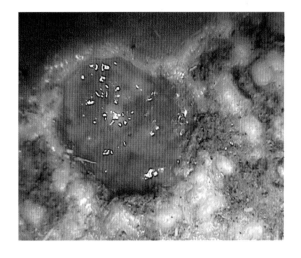

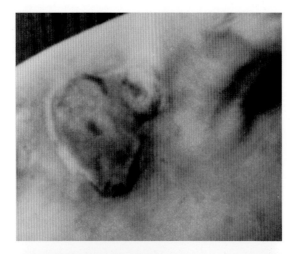

75-YEAR OLD WOMAN WITH CANCER "CAUSED BY NUCLEAR TESTING IN NEVADA." THE REACTION IS TO A SINGLE APPLICATION OF A COMPOUND X PASTE, APPLIED TO AN AREA ABOUT 3 CENTIMETERS IN DIAMETER. AS SEEN, THE REACTION OCCURRED IN A MUCH LARGER REGION. THE ESCHAR GIVES THE APPEARANCE OF CHARRED TISSUE.

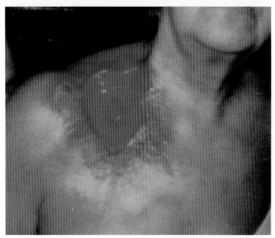

THIS PHOTO, SCANNED FROM A VERY OLD POLAROID, SHOWS THE AREA AFTER DETACH-MENT OF THE ESCHAR, AN EVENT THAT OCCURS ABOUT 12-16 DAYS AFTER USE OF SUCH PASTES. NOTE THAT THERE WAS NO DAMAGE TO BLOOD VESSELS

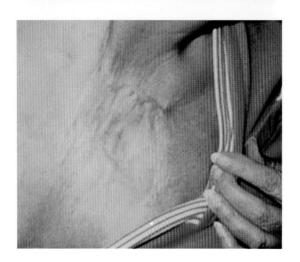

THIS PICTURE WAS TAKEN A YEAR AFTER THE TREATMENT WAS COMPLETED. THE PATIENT IS NOW 94 YEARS OF AGE AND COMPLAINS OCCASIONALLY OF SLIGHT ITCHINESS IN THE SCAR TISSUE LEFT AFTER USE OF THE BLOOD-ROOT PASTE. SHE HAS HAD NO RECURRENCE.

BASAL CELL CARCINOMA ON RIGHT UPPER
CHEST OF 74-YEAR OLD MAN. HE USED A
BLOODROOT PASTE. THE PICTURE SHOWS THE
FORMATION OF THE ESCHAR AND INFLAMMA-
TION SURROUNDING THE TREATMENT SITE.

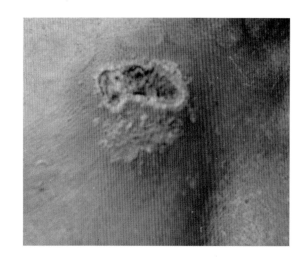

NOTE THAT THE ESCHAR IS DARKER AND
THICKER AND THAT IT IS BEGINNING TO PULL
AWAY FROM THE EDGES. THE SURROUNDING
AREA IS INFLAMED, A REACTION TYPICAL OF
BLOODROOT PASTES.

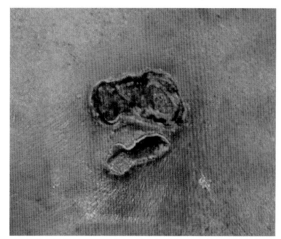

THIS PICTURE SHOWS THE SITE AFTER MOST OF
THE ESCHAR HAS DETACHED. NOTE THAT THE
INFLAMMATION HAS SUBSIDED AND THE SITE
ITSELF IS CLEAN EXCEPT FOR SOME REMAINING
ESCHAR (ON THE LOWER EDGE OF THE LARGER
CRATER.) THE PATIENT TREATED HIMSELF SIX
YEARS AGO FOR THIS CONDITION AS WELL AS
ANOTHER ON HIS LEG. HE IS NOW 80 YEARS
OLD AND WELL.

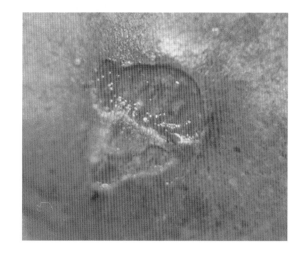

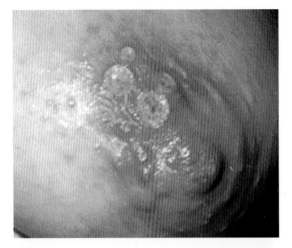

IDEAL RESPONSE. THE PATIENT BEGAN WITH A CONVENTIONAL BLOODROOT PASTE. SHE COULD NOT TOLERATE THE PAIN AND SWITCHED TO THE AUTHOR'S ENUCLEATING SALVE ON THE SECOND DAY. SHE ADDED TINY AMOUNTS OF THE BLACK PASTE TO MAKE THE PREPARATION PENETRATE.

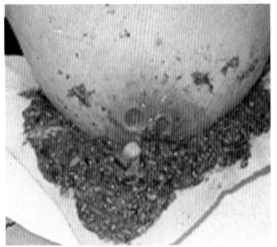

DAY 9. THE PATIENT DISCHARGED A NUMBER OF SIMILAR MASSES, SEVERAL OF THEM LARGER THAN THE ONE SHOWN. THE PICTURE SHOWS ONE OF THE SMALLER MASSES THAT FELL ONTO THE POULTICE WHEN THE DRESSING WAS CHANGED. THE POULTICE WAS USED ONCE THE ESCHARS (SHOWN ABOVE) DETACHED AND THE SITE WAS OPEN.

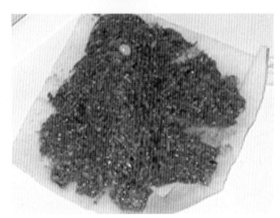

MASS ON POULTICE.

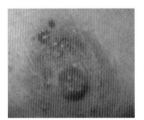

DAY 29.
THE AREA HEALED ALMOST PERFECTLY.

CHAPTER 11

Answers to Questions

The simple answer is: it depends on you. Many people have followed the instructions that sometimes come with the salves; others have been directed by friends familiar with the salves. Some will find the information in this book sufficient. A few have ordered the salves and not used them because they were uncertain as to how to start and what to expect. If you can find someone who has used them before, you will feel more comfortable. If you know a nurse, doctor, or other health care practitioner willing to assist you, this may enhance your confidence a bit. In researching this book, I kept finding more and more people who used the salves without any supervision. They were quite secure in their understanding of what to do and what to anticipate. However, I also spoke with people who failed to remove their tumors properly, usually because they were uncertain as to how to proceed.

Perhaps the better answer is that relatively small tumors that are on the surface of the skin or close to the surface can be treated with a minimal amount of supervision. Larger and deeper tumors should most often be treated by those experienced in the use of the salves.

2. HOW MUCH DO THE SALVES COST?

This varies according to the product, quantity purchased, and the supplier. There are truly a large number of escharotic salves on the market, and they are bottled in quantities as small as a fraction of an ounce (enough for a small basal cell carcinoma or Kaposi's sarcoma lesion) to two-ounce jars, which often sell for less than the smaller bottles. Moreover, producers have different pricing arrangements, reflecting either their costs or what they consider the value of their product is to the patient. A few producers supply their products on a "love offering" basis, with a suggested minimum for those who can afford to pay and free to those who cannot. Some companies also have an unlimited money-back guarantee if the product fails to work. In 1998, most escharotic salves were priced around thirty to fifty dollars, regardless of the amount of salve contained in the jar. Since larger tumors require more salve, patients with such tumors can consider asking the producers to supply their product in four-ounce to one pound jars.

In addition to the escharotic salve, there may be a need for poulticing. Though the ingredients for poultices are quite inexpensive, larger and deeper tumors may require more poulticing, perhaps two to three months of treatment. Then, there is need for a drawing and/or a healing salve and eventually perhaps an ointment for scar removal. In all, the total expense for all these products will probably be more than one hundred dollars, but it depends, of course, on the actual products used and the amount required. Persons using the salve are advised to pay attention to when their supply is running low and to reorder at least ten days before running out.

Most patients report that the cost of bandages far exceeded the cost of the salves. Though self-adhering bandages, such as Tegaderm™, are by far the least stressful and most convenient to use, they are expensive. Some patients therefore use thin plastic such as sandwich bags. The disadvantages of such "bandages" are that they do not contain the salve as well and patients often have tape marks or allergic reactions where adhesives were used to secure the plastic. Though these marks and irritations eventually disappear, they can be annoying.

Over and above these costs, patients should factor in the cost of adjunctive treatments. These are well advised regardless of whether or not the escharotics are used.

3. What if I get an adverse reaction to the tape?

Most patients eventually become very sensitive or allergic to the tape used for bandaging. Often, the skin where the tape was applied remains irritated long after the drama of the salve use has subsided. If using a self-adhering bandage, it may be necessary to change to some other bandaging method. One way to avoid such reactions is to change the shape and size of the bandages used. By rotating the position and switching sizes, the tape can be placed on different areas of the skin. With a little practice, most sites permit quite a few variations and give relief to areas that are becoming too reactive. Some people develop a partiality to particular brands of tape; others find that changing brands now and then offers a respite.

If none of these methods work, it may be possible to apply beeswax to gauze or cloth and to hold the bandage in place by wrapping the site. Breast cancer patients may be able to achieve this through use of an athletic bra, but the risk of the escharotic spreading is greater when the area immediately surrounding the treatment site is not protected from contact with the escharotic. Coating the area outside the designated treatment site with something waxy or oily sometimes works. It goes without saying that if an aggressive escharotic spreads, the reactive area may be larger and the patient will suffer more than necessary.

4. How long will it take for the salve to work?

Every tumor and every patient is different. Much depends on the type of salve used, how aggressively it is used, and the size, type, and depth of the tumor. Which technique is used also affects treatment time. Some patients with Kaposi's sarcoma lesions (an opportunistic cancerous condition associated primarily with AIDS) have had growths fall off in three to five days. A few other skin cancers have also responded this quickly, but some tumors take much longer, especially when the salve is applied too thinly. As a general rule, it takes roughly two weeks for the eschar to detach. Then, depending on the method of treatment, another round or two of treatment may be necessary. For planning purposes, it is probably best to assume that a deep breast tumor may require two to six months of treatment unless scratches or incisions have been made in the eschar to promote more complete penetration of the tumor during the initial treatment.

5. What about bleeding?

Unless the area where the salve is applied is accidentally struck fairly roughly, use of the salve is not normally attended by bleeding. However, just as a scab will bleed if bumped or if pulled off prematurely, bleeding can occur at the treatment site if the area is stressed. When this does happen, seldom is more than a drop or two of blood lost. In somewhat isolated situations, the drawing action of the tallow-based salves may break tiny blood vessels near the skin; but even in such instances, bleeding is normally minimal.

As a precautionary measure, it is suggested that patients keep a bottle of *Yunnan Paiyao*[76] on hand. This is a Chinese herbal remedy for bleeding. The bottle contains one tiny pill (often almost invisibly buried in the cotton at the top of the bottle) that can be taken orally in the case of bleeding or hemorrhaging and a powder that can be applied externally (or taken internally with warm water). These precautions are especially important where there is already a tendency for an ulcerated area to bleed even before use of the salve or when angiogenesis exists. If Yunnan Paiyao is not available, turmeric powder, or cayenne can be used to arrest bleeding. Besides stopping bleeding, turmeric is antiseptic and antitumoral. Turmeric can also be taken internally—in food, capsules, tablets, and/or honey.

6. Can I get the area wet?

Since moisture will dilute the salve and cause it to spread, it is recommended that the treatment area be kept completely dry, at least once the crack has formed. Depending on the type of bandage used, it may be possible to bathe without water leaking into the treatment site. It is usually advisable to keep the bandage on when bathing or showering and to change the dressing immediately after the bath or shower. This is especially the case when the opening is suppurating (discharging pus and other materials).

Early in the treatment as well as once the area starts to heal, the bandage can be removed before bathing as long as the water is safe and a clean dressing is applied immediately afterwards.

7. What if the escharotic salve does accidentally smear?

Wipe off the excess as soon as possible. If the salve has already caused the area to blister, cover it with a thin layer of the healing salve or a mixture of turmeric, goldenseal, and calendula oil to keep it antiseptic and prevent infection. Though it may be challenging, try not to include this area in the airtight bandage.

8. Do you have any suggestions for bandaging?

Unwanted spread of the salve can be prevented by (1) placing paper tape with a mild adhesive coating around the designated application site. This enables the adhesive bandage to contact the paper tape without affecting containment of the escharotic. Alternatively, (2) the area can be covered with an ointment such as Unpetroleum Jelly™ or a mixture of beeswax and olive oil. This will prevent a self-adhering bandage from fitting tightly around the escharotic, but it will offer some protection to the surrounding area. Another method is (3) to cut a hole the size of the tumor in an adhesive bandage, adhere it to the skin, apply the salve through the hole, and cover this with another bandage. The advantage of this method is that the self-adhering bandage can be left in place for a longer period of time. This is less traumatic to the surrounding skin, but it does

not permit the skin to breathe quite as much, and it tends to aggravate the tendencies towards allergic reactions to the adhesives.

9. How many times should I reapply the salve?

The proper answer to this question is that it depends on the size of the tumor, its depth (beneath the surface of the skin), the particular product used, the method used, reactivity to the salve, and the appearance of the site when the eschar detaches. One time is sometimes sufficient, but there is no specific minimum or maximum number of applications of this salve.

Salve producers have various suggestions, but some of the escharotics are so aggressive that they will cause a reaction in healthy as well as malignant tissue. This is therefore a feature of that particular escharotic so that, despite claims to the contrary, reactions are not a clue to malignancy or lack thereof. Some patients are timid and apply the salve too thinly. They interpret the mild reaction in a diagnostic fashion that is probably not correct. Others are using a mild escharotic on a deep tumor so that reactions are necessarily slow since contact with the tumor may not occur on the first application.

Thus, the answer to this question is probably that no determinations are possible until the eschar detaches. At this time, site inspection will determine whether or not to continue use of the escharotic or enucleating salve. Only when the area is very clean, when no evidence of any tumor remains, is the escharotic process complete.

10. Do you have any suggestions for how to inspect the site for residual malignancy?

Though examination of the site after detachment of the eschar is no doubt the most important step in the entire salve process, it is not easy for inexperienced persons to identify what they see. Magnifying glasses and high resolution close up photographs make the viewing a little easier. Digital cameras facilitate the examination of enlargements on the computer monitor within seconds after taking the picture; and these images are often clearer than what one sees when looking directly at the site.

11. What happens if terminating the treatment too soon?

If malignancy is allowed to remain in the area, the tumor may grow and/or metastasize. The site should therefore not be allowed to close before all malignancy is removed. Moreover, in addition to the issue of leaving some of the tumor in the body, it should be pointed out that when the area is not healthy, excessive amounts of scar tissue are likely to form. Use of an escharotic at a future date will be impaired by the resistance of the scar tissue to penetration by the paste (or salves).

Because of the sensitivity of the site, patients are often deeply afraid to reapply the escharotic after the eschar detaches. It is at this time that an adequate pain control program is imperative. In general, more relief is conferred by pain relievers mixed into the salve than by use of topical analgesics.

Once the tumor is exposed, direct contact with it is possible. This allows milder products to be quite effective as part of the pain is caused by reactions with healthy tissue that has to be destroyed in order to reach the tumor. The escharotic or enucleating salve can either be painted directly onto the tumor or a milder product can be gently packed into the crater.

Second and third eschars will usually form faster and detach sooner than the original eschar. If no reaction to the escharotic takes place, further external use will be of no avail. However, it is important to determine why the reaction did not occur: (1) no malignancy remains, (2) the escharotic did not make proper contact with the tumor, or (3) scar tissue or other impediments prevented a reaction from occurring.

12. If there is no reaction, does it mean that there is no cancer in the body?

This question was partially answered in the previous reply. Since not all producers divulge the contents of their products, it is difficult to know whether the escharotic is self-biopsying, as many claim, or high in zinc chloride or other substances that burn. If the product is primarily herbal and alkaloidal, chances are that an absence of a reaction means either that all the malignancy has been destroyed or that what remains is very deep and that further use for two or three days may produce a reaction.

In some instances, patients have had allopathic treatments that walled off the tumor area to prevent spread of the malignancy to other parts of the body. In these cases, the salve seems unable to penetrate or cross the barrier. Applying the salve to a second site may then bring about a reaction even when none occurred during the first application.

13. IS THERE A DANGER OF THE CANCER SPREADING BY USE OF THE SALVES?

Though there is no general consensus on this question, the proper answer is probably that it depends on several factors: the amount of inflammation, the extent of the increase in circulation, and the rapidity of the process. The danger is not necessarily any greater than with biopsy procedures or surgery, but it exists. If the process is aborted, it is likely that any part of the tumor that was not necrotized will be stimulated by the irritation to the area. Careful technique ought to reduce most of the risk.

14. WILL THERE BE SCARRING?

Some say "always" and others say "usually." Some people have almost imperceptible scars and others more significant marks. It is difficult to say why some people scar and others do not. One hypothesis is that where there is infection at the tumor site, there is more likelihood of scarring. Careful use of poultices seems to reduce scarring as well as to promote healthy granulation of new tissue. However, much may depend on individual tendencies to scar, skin types, fatty deposits, and the type of salve used. In any event, the amount of scarring that does occur varies enormously from person to person. It is generally less than that left by surgery, but more varied in pattern.

In a few instances, the marks left by the tape are larger than the scars, but the tape marks do eventually disappear whereas the scars will not vanish on their own. Internal and external consumption of turmeric reduces scarring. This can be commenced at the beginning of treatment or used years later; its effect is quite gradual. I have spoken to a few producers of the salve to see if they would consider adding turmeric to their products, particularly to the healing salve. At least one salve does now contain turmeric; its producer reported that complaints of scarring have declined significantly since the change in the formula.

After the salve process is completely finished, patients can try a product called *Scargo*, a blend of oils described by Edgar Cayce in his readings,[77] and/or *Vicco Vanishing Cream*, a turmeric ointment from India. Red clover combination tea, tincture, capsules, syrup, or ointment may, in some cases, also help to reduce scar tissue if used regularly for many months. Specific scar removal products are listed on the Web site: http://www.cancer-salves.com.

15. CAN THE SALVES PREVENT RECURRENCES?

Just as surgery and other standard cancer treatments do not prevent the recurrence of cancer, the salves also are not preventative. Their successful use in no way precludes a recurrence. However, many people routinely reapply the salves at six- to twelve-month intervals just to see if there is a reaction. They regard the absence of a reaction as good news: i.e., the cancer has not come back.

Since the salves are not a substitute for other diagnostic procedures, I cannot speak for the reliability of this practice except to note that many who do vouch for it maintain that they regard such routine use of the salve as a satisfactory prophylactic measure.

On the opposite side of this debate, it may be noted that everyone has heard of cancers that were not detected by standard means as well as lumps that were blithely regarded as innocent and dismissed without tests to prove such. If someone were to apply the salves as some sort of diagnostic test after being assured that there is no cause for alarm, some extra satisfaction might be gained or valuable time not wasted in false complacency.

16. How long should salve use be continued?

Basically this process requires consistency. If use of the products is discontinued before all the cancer has been removed, there is virtually no doubt but that the cancer that remains will proliferate—and necessitate some procedure for dealing with the remaining malignancy.

Historically, there has been debate as to whether to use a relatively aggressive paste and deal with the malignancy faster or a gentler product that takes more time. I believe that the more aggressive pastes require supervision and serious pain management. Moreover, there is some risk that the massive inflammation caused by such methods could disseminate the tumor.

There is also likely to be more scarring when the major function of the paste is to burn the tumor. Milder products take longer, often many months. Even when patients are fed up with the process, few choose to speed up the tumor removal by going with a more aggressive escharotic or having surgery.

17. Is there anything I should do after discontinuing use of the salve?

The skin may be tender for some time. One patient recommended treating the area with a cream or flax seed oil until all hypersensitivity is gone. Another suggested using a thin layer of a healing salve without bandaging. Yet another used a homeopathic arnica ointment. Mixing the Vicco cream with Christopher's *Red Sun Balm* is another possibility as is Hildegard's violet salve. The object at this time is to reduce scarring and "catch" any residual, however microscopic it may be. Care should be taken to avoid everything but the highest quality and freshest oils since free radicals are present in many oils. Ointments that stimulate growth of tissue should not be used until the entire malignancy has been destroyed since premature use of such products could conceivably promote proliferation of malignant cells.

18. Can the salves be used by people who have already had surgery or other allopathic treatments?

Generally the answer to this question is "yes." Moreover, when there are questions as to whether or not the entire malignancy was removed or whether it is recurring, it is often maintained that, for safe measure, the salves or some milder anticancer ointment can be used post-surgically to destroy whatever was missed in surgery as well as whatever might have returned. For such purposes, a mild, "self-biopsying" salve can be considered.

19. How long after discontinuing use of the salve should I continue using the internal herbs?

A correct reply to this question demands knowledge of the real condition of the person. A broad answer would be that patients with a history of cancer might take a prophylactic dosage of herbs for at least six months to a year after all clinical signs of cancer have disappeared. After this, periodic preventative regimes may be wise. These might include such things as juice fasting, saunas, and a maintenance or a preventative dosage of herbs for at least three weeks every spring and/or fall.

If there is such a thing as a cancer temperament or predisposition to cancer, then sound preventative measures are essential: just as a diabetic should avoid sugar and only eat foods that do not aggravate blood sugar levels, people who have had cancer should adopt sound programs for maintaining health.

20. What about diet?

It makes good sense to be aware of the role of nutrition in health. The body is organic and can only be regenerated through the ingestion of organic foods and herbs. Even if some medical or catalytic benefit is claimed for inorganic substances, they cannot be used by the body to rebuild tissues.

There are aspects of a proper diet that make perfect sense for everyone, regardless of whether or not they ever had cancer. For example, complete elimination of refined sugar and flour from the diet is advisable. Avoidance of other processed and refined foods is also recommended. Reliance on as much organically grown foods as possible is also sound practice. Also, no food should be microwaved!

Ideally, diets should be individually tailored to each patient. Those with good appetites and digestion can allow themselves a wider array of food. Those who have poor appetites, weak digestion, bouts of nausea, bloating and gas, or who tend to form mucus easily should remain careful for at least two years after all signs of illness have gone. The symptoms just mentioned are indicative of poor digestion. Until the metabolism is balanced, care should be exercised in the choice and preparation of food. For some people, it takes several years to achieve optimum health, whereas others may only be able to avert chronic disease by learning to manage the idiosyncrasies of their particular bodies. In any event, it pays to watch the diet and to decline foods that are difficult to digest.[78]

21. Where can I get answers to questions not covered here?

Send an e-mail over the author's Web site: http://www.cancersalves.com and look for the answer in two or three days.

CHAPTER 12

Boluses

DR. JOHN CHRISTOPHER used herbal pessaries and suppositories to treat gynecological, prostate, and colon conditions. His theory was that just as poor soil attracts pests, tumors survive in morbid environments where they feed on compromised tissues. Like many natural healers, Christopher believed that malignancy thrives where there is toxicity and a deprivation of nutrients crucial to the health of normal tissue. He believed that cysts and tumors are scavengers and that, to the extent that the conditions that sustain the growths are not corrected, disease cannot be cured. His treatments were therefore designed to remove toxicity and nourish healthy tissues so that the body could reject the disease and the patient be restored to health. For this purpose, he developed herbal boluses, large pills that are inserted vaginally or rectally, to correct the underlying conditions. The herbs used in his boluses are neutralizing to toxins, absorbent, and nourishing to tissues with the potential for health. In his experience, tumors either broke

down and were discharged from the body via the normal eliminatory channels, or they separated from the healthy tissue when deprived of the morbid matter on which they had been sustained. In this latter case, they would be expelled, vaginally or rectally.

Christopher reported a case of a spider-like tumor the size of a half-dollar that dropped out the very day the woman suffering from this condition had decided to give up on herbal approaches. He also described cases of severe deterioration of internal organs that were completely resolved by the use of suppositories.

In his philosophy, the terrain was everything: change the environment and the conditions existing in that environment will necessarily also change. Christopher's bolus may or may not work precisely as he described—there does not seem to be a way to determine this—but satisfaction with the use of this simple bolus approaches 100 percent. Weeks before press time, the daughter of the owner of a health foods store used the bolus for five days and passed a mass the size of a tennis ball. She was astounded, and, of course, pleased. Others with yeast infections, vaginitis, hyperplasia, dysplasia, cervical cancer, or a history of vaginal discharges, itchiness, or discomfort have used the suppositories with remarkable success and relief. In fact, these simple boluses might be Nature's gift to women.

So far as colon-rectal cancer or cancer of the male reproductive system are concerned, I only personally know of one person who used Christopher's boluses for such purposes. He combined many therapies and told me that the mass had become softer but had not disappeared entirely. Eventually, he had the tumor removed using the Mohs method which, interestingly, he did not realize relied on an escharotic. He has been completely well since.

Another person related a case to me that sounds much like what Christopher mentioned. This man expelled a tumor the size of a small turnip after internal consumption of a Compound X formula and a bout of diarrhea. He did not use any herbal suppositories. The tumor did have thread-like protrusions similar to the spider-like mass described by Christopher in his lectures. Though this lends credence to Christopher's report, verifiable cures of colon cancer attributed to use of herbal boluses have yet to be reported to me.

The Bolus

The bolus contains equal parts of eight common herbs that are readily available: squaw vine herb, slippery elm bark, yellow dock root, comfrey root, marshmallow root, chickweed herb, goldenseal root, and mullein leaves.[79] Cocoa butter is used as a base. Variations of this formula have been reported; but, as Christopher originally described it, the formula seems effective for many gynecological conditions.

The boluses are inserted vaginally or rectally, as indicated. Sanitary napkins or panty liners are used to protect clothing and bedding. The number of suppositories used and the length of time necessary for healing seems to differ from person to person. Much depends on the extent of the infection or malignancy and the responsiveness of the patient. A few patients have used one bolus every other day for two weeks. Others have used one or two a day for weeks or months, even three-to-six months.

Christopher recommended that use of the bolus be accompanied by vaginal douches and/or colon enemas before insertion of a new bolus. He provided several formulae for decocting strong teas using distilled water.[80] Patients were instructed to place about $\frac{1}{4}$ to $\frac{1}{2}$ cup of the tea—reduced to body temperature—in a syringe and to insert the decoction as appropriate, preferably while reclining on a slant board. Christopher said that the treatment would be even more effective if the abdominal region is gently massaged while the fluid is retained.

Christopher recommended that the suppositories be used for uterine cysts and tumors as well as virtually all problems of the male reproductive system and eliminatory system. He believed that the herbs work more or less systemically, that they are absorbed by the body where they spread throughout the reproductive, urinary, and eliminatory systems. Once circulated in the body, the herbs function like a sponge and begin absorbing toxins, acid wastes, and abnormal growths. The detoxifying effect ends in the removal of morbid conditions in the reproductive and eliminatory systems. However, there is a tonifying action in addition to the cleansing; the second function of the bolus herbs is to nourish nutrient deficient tissues and support regeneration of compromised systems of the body.

Since herbal nutrients are absorbed into the blood stream, Christopher regarded their action as more systemic than local. Even the lymphatic system is thought to be stimulated by use of the boluses with the recommended teas, douches, and enemas. A few people using the suppositories reported no discharge at all. This suggests that their bodies did, in fact, absorb not only the herbs but the cocoa butter as well. In most cases, however, discharge did occur.

As noted, I only know one person who used herbal boluses for a malignant colon condition. I know another person who used them for less than a week when told she had cervical cancer. Six years earlier, she had had an abnormal Pap smear, but had ignored the advice of her gynecologist and failed to have her condition checked at the recommended intervals. When she did finally bite the bullet, the news alarmed her. The Pap smear was followed by a cone biopsy that revealed the presence of cancerous cells. She went into gear immediately: she flew out to see Michio Kushi of macrobiotic fame, began use of the vaginal suppositories, and took many herbs internally.

This mother of two had been informed that her chances of dealing with the condition surgically were excellent. She wanted however, to avoid surgery. She used the bolus for six days before deciding that her need "to play it safe" dictated a hysterectomy. She therefore submitted to the operation, but when the uterus and cervix were removed, no cancer was found.

This isolated incident neither proves nor disproves that the suppositories worked. The cancer could have been misdiagnosed; the pathologists may have failed to find remaining malignancy in the tissue samples they studied. However, there may have been cancer, and the condition may have been cured in the brief time she allowed herself to experiment with alternatives.

Unlike the salves, I do not feel there is much anecdotal or clinical evidence for use of the suppositories with malignant conditions—neither is there reason to discount Christopher's experience. There is simply a need for more information, more reporting of experience, and more study. I suspect, however, that use would have to be consistent for a considerable time period before relief would be measurable.

Other Gynecological Conditions

Many people using the suppositories for candida albicans have in fact reported a feeling of comfort they had not previously known. A few described increased initial itchiness and then less than usual distress after the first two or three days. There is no adequate way to determine how pervasive the effects of the herbs are; patients measure results by how they feel: less itchy, more ease, less discharge, no odor.

Rather remarkable results have been reported to me concerning the use of boluses for other vaginal and cervical conditions:[81] various dysplasias and hyperplasias. In these cases, considerable improvement was reported with fairly brief use, one-to-three months. It should, however, be mentioned that chlorophyll suppositories and douches are also often equally effective.

Christopher said that the boluses can be used for uterine cysts and fibroids as well as malignant tumors. Though I only know of one such case, I do not discredit the information since I have also heard of similar success stories using large capsules containing black strap molasses.[82] In these cases, the growths did separate and fall out. Different formulae could very likely have comparable effects. More investigation of the herbal boluses seems the only way to determine the appropriate circumstances for their use.

Decades before Christopher, Dr. Eli G. Jones used suppositories for rectal cancer. Two of his formulas are reported in chapter 8 (see page 114). I do not know anyone who has used either of these preparations, but both doctors used cocoa butter as a base for the herbs. If interested in using such suppositories, be careful to use good cocoa butter, not a product that has become rancid. Also keep in mind that the boluses are to be used in conjunction with douches or enemas as well as herbal teas. These supportive formulae help to flush out toxins, restore hormonal balance, and boost immune function.

At this juncture, I have no doubts whatsoever but that the boluses are an excellent treatment for many conditions of the reproductive and eliminatory systems. I simply do not know that they resolve malignancy—nor that they fail to do so. As such, I regard the use of such boluses as a sensible approach to conditions that may benefit by this particular method of delivery of herbs to places where needed—even if the function is more palliative that curative.

Finally, there is one remedy that I know has relieved distress caused by irradiation. This is the use of slightly warm unrefined sesame oil douches or enemas, daily for three weeks. This simple treatment seems to restore elasticity to tissue that has been burned. It also relieves much of the pain caused by dryness—and it restores libido. Taking daily baths in water containing half a cup of baking soda and half a cup of sea salt also draws radiation out of the body and promotes relaxation. This should be continued for three weeks (or every other day for six weeks). Stay in the tub for twenty to thirty minutes.

CHAPTER 13

Health

ESPITE NEW TECHNOLOGY that permits earlier diagnosis than in previous times, cancer often has a serious foothold in the body before it is discovered. Moreover, even with the alleged benefits of commencing treatment at a much less advanced stage of the disease, modern medicine has not appreciably extended survival time.

In the first chapter, it was noted that cancer has been found in the remains of dinosaurs and mummies. The search for a reliable treatment must therefore be almost as old as Time.

As we have seen, escharotics methods are ancient. They were typically used after tumors had become conspicuous by virtue of their size or ulceration. As such, the success of these treatments relative to surgery, chemotherapy, and radiation seems worthy of more than a cursory review. Several people have said that after learning about these older strategies for dealing with cancer, they were no longer afraid of the disease. While knowing about botanical treatments does confer a measure of peace of mind, the truth is no one wants to have cancer.

DATA

There is no data to support the belief that longevity is greater using some sort of escharotic or enucleating treatment in combination with internal tonics instead of the protocols that are today standard—nor, of course, is there data confirming the opposite view. The arguments for or against one or the other strategy for treating cancer are thus partly subjective: botanical treatments appeal to the desire to be more in harmony with Nature whereas modern medicine may claim to be more aligned with science. Neither approach is infallible. No matter how we look at the situation, people do die of cancer or the side effects of cancer and/or its treatment—though this said, unlike surgery and chemotherapy, medical doctors, ancient and contemporary, vehemently deny that there are any deaths directly attributable to escharotic use. This said, there are, of course, people for whom these products were either used too late or for whom they failed to work.

Since there are also those who were cured by internal tonics alone, it is always worth considering these and holding the external measures in reserve for future use in case a bolder attack on the cancer is required.

The pastes and salves are used to destroy tumorous growths, but the internal remedies restore health to the vital organs of the body and promote proper detoxification while simultaneously helping to eliminate cancer. The herbs used to treat the disease from within are not covered sufficiently in this book, but it should be understood that the tonics are multi-purpose.

ACUTE VERSUS CHRONIC DISEASES

No one knows exactly what cancer is. It may be a collection of conditions that share certain common denominators, one being somewhat below normal metabolic functioning. Metabolism may be impaired, as Jones thought, by excessive immunization and poor dietary habits. Predisposition can also be genetic, environmental, temperamental—or any combination of the foregoing.

Most people who have cancer do not throw off illnesses well. Many patients were probably chronically ill for years before the diagnosis of cancer, but they were so asymptomatic that they thought they were enjoying better health than others. However, the failure to react to infections and other insults demanding acute responses is indicative of compromised immunity and a host of other problems that all need to be addressed before deep and genuine health can be experienced.

A good treatment program should address both the underlying weaknesses as well as the malignancy. This is the purpose of the tonics and adjunctive measures used by holistic practitioners in the past and present. Most oncologists as well as patients are deeply focused on cancer, but the fact is that patients usually die of complications, not the cancer itself. A sensible protocol ought to take the patient and the patient's overall health as seriously as the cancer.

This said, there is no one tonic or pill that is right for everyone. Unlike the external preparations, the internal remedies are tailored more to the specific needs of the individual. Certainly, there are some standard elixirs like the *trifolium compound* (a tonic based on red clover) that have been supplied to thousands of patients regardless of symptoms. However, individual needs are better addressed by reference to the particular constitutional weaknesses of the person. Qualified herbalists are generally able to recommend herbs or combinations of herbs that are suitable for various conditions, but they tend to be less comfortable working with cancer than the overall health picture.

In appendix B, a large number of Dr. John Christopher's formulae are given. He, above all others, worked in an organ specific manner. His understanding of health is made clear by his statement that one should not blame flies for the garbage but rather garbage for the flies. He saw cancer as a scavenger that cleaned up the terrain. His remedies therefore address the terrain.

For those people who have never missed a day of work, who have not come down with colds and viral infections when "the bugs have been going around," it is very difficult to understand that they are ill with a life-threatening disease. However, when the constitutional idiosyncrasies that relate to cancer are explained, patients realize that it is not actually healthy to be so free of symptoms, that it is generally better to run a fever now and then and to allow the body to function with a little more short-term risk so as to avoid developing a chronic condition, one characterized by various levels of morbidity—and deterioration of the terrain. When the issues of internal well being are related to overall health, almost everyone is able to see ways to improve everything from eating habits to life styles.

DEFERRED ISSUES

Cancer may be a disease of deferred issues. Not only have immune responses been depressed, but emotional reactions are also often denied or delayed as are matters of the heart and soul. These subjective matters are treated as though subordinate to other priorities, ones usually governed by outer concerns such as responsibilities, success, and the goals the mind sets that operate against personal happiness. To the extent that the disease calls attention to the deferred needs of the inner being, it is friend. A suitable healing plan must incorporate the need for dealing directly with malignancy, the underlying causes of malignancy and inherent weaknesses of the constitution, and the need for movement of all the suppressed responses.

STAGNATION OF ENERGY

If the hypothesis that cancer patients have systems of the body that are not operating at peak efficiency is accepted, then there are logical ways to pursue relief from disease. Chinese medicine uses the term "stagnation of energy." This is a useful image to hold when trying to understand the benefits of moving the stagnation. Western natural medicine speaks of blockages in much the same way that Oriental medicine refers to stagnation; and Ayurveda, the traditional system of medicine from India, refers to *ama*, essentially a metabolic residual that clogs and obstructs the flow of energy.

For years prior to the detection of malignancy, most cancer patients suffered from some level of digestive, eliminatory, and/or lymphatic stagnation. Since problems in these systems of the body do not interfere in any significant way with outer functioning, they are not regarded as medical issues. However, they are the precursors to chronic illness.

Natural medicine is thus concerned with all types of congestion: in the form of mucus, phlegm, and catarrh as well as deposits in the arteries and lower intestines. Many practitioners of holistic medicine insist that without decongestion of the bowels, no real healing is possible. In my experience, good health depends on proper digestion, assimilation, and elimination. Without good digestion and assimilation, the nutrient value of food is wasted and regeneration of compromised tissues and systems of the body cannot occur. Since assimilation of nutrients takes place in the small and large intestines as well as the stomach, tissues will be deprived so long as any part of the gastrointestinal tract is malfunctioning.

DETOXIFICATION AND TONIFICATION

We live in a time of unparalleled pollution and adulteration of our food and water supply. Survival of the fittest and good health may depend on periodic detoxification as well as adequate efforts to regenerate damaged tissues.

Detoxification is a technical term referring to measures that relieve the body of chemical toxicity as well as surfeit, metabolic residuals that are deposited in various parts of the body where they congest those areas. There are many ways to purify the body, ranging from fasting to specific dietary regimes and herbal remedies to medical protocols. The simplest involve modest improvements in the diet and supplements that cleanse the blood and liver, improve elimination, and relieve lymphatic stagnation. The most complex entail the removal of parasites and serious contaminants such as mercury and lead. While it may be possible to overcome cancer without addressing digestion and elimination as well as the functioning of the liver and blood stream, kidneys, and bowels, it hardly seems realistic to

expect health without attention to the overall condition of the body.

Tonification is another technical term. In essence, it refers to those strategies that correct deficiency conditions. Detoxification and tonification employ different diets and herbs because detoxification removes unwanted substances from the body whereas tonification rebuilds depleted systems of the body. Since every cell has a different normal life before it is replaced, each system of the body is rebuilt at its own pace.

RESPONSE RATES

Immune stimulation may occur within minutes of taking an immune boosting herb or supplement. Dark field microscopy will then reveal increased white blood cell activity. As the white blood cells become more efficient, debris in the lymph, infections in the blood, and deformities in red blood cells are transformed. Patients feel better almost immediately, but this does not mean healing is complete.

Likewise, digestion and elimination are often improved with one meal. What this means is that if someone is used to eating indigestible or almost indigestible food, a single meal of wholesome food that is prepared properly will prove that bloating and discomfort after eating is not necessary. It does not, however, mean that the side effects of years of poor food have been resolved. It may take months to tonify the lower intestine and two years to regenerate the liver. Still, so long as new insults are not added to the existing injuries, most people will feel that they are on a valid healing path.

Ultimately, many will desire a level of health that is today rare on the Planet. They may wish to antidote vaccines and medications that were given to them in the name of health but that, in fact, compromised the integrity of their bodies. There are remedies for this, but they should be prescribed by experts who understand their proper use.

The Healing Path

A remarkably clairvoyant *kahuna* in Hawaii once told me that, at the subconscious level, people resist whatever does not feel good. Morrnah Simeona suggested that real healing does not take place if the threshold where resistance is met is crossed. Since I had for so long been convinced that all real healing had to feel good, Morrnah's words made me question the salves. I was reluctant to cop out by saying that the ends justify the means, that the salve is the lesser of two evils. I struggled to develop a method that was more tolerable; however, I have yet to find a totally painless way to remove a malignant mass.

The internal tonics can indeed be effective; and since they are more systemic in action than the salves, they are perhaps the closest I have found to a tolerable treatment for cancer. There are, of course, more esoteric techniques that do not employ any physical means at all. I have been honored to have witnessed a few spontaneous remissions, enough to realize that there is much to the healing process that has yet to be recognized as significant.

The problem is that people have been taught to think of their diseases as physical and several patients have said that while they recognize they fit the psychological profile of a cancer patient to a "T," they prefer to predicate their cure on something physical rather than metaphysical.

As such, the love-hate relationship to the salves can be accepted until something better is found to replace the escharotic and enucleating methods.

There are invisible functions that the salves perform that have earned the respect of most people who used them. Cancer cells are not just malignant, but highly toxic. When they die, they put pressure on the body to dispose of toxic debris. The symptoms of the die off can vary from fatigue to achiness to somewhat severe grouchiness and an ashen cast to the skin. By creating a safety-valve for the discharge of morbid material, the internal systems of the body are spared much of the burden of detoxification. Most people experience this relief as an increase in vitality and alertness. Many felt that they suddenly became more intelligent.

It is doubtful that anyone actually becomes more intelligent, but it is entirely possible that people who are less compromised by toxicity are better able to demonstrate their innate potential. With the internal tonics, these subtle improvements in perception are less dramatic. This is probably easily explained by the fact that the toxicity does have to handled internally so that the quantum leaps in awareness are achieved several months later than when the external treatments are used.

When expressing my reservations to patients, I was surprised by their comments. Most gave me answers I had not anticipated. They were not concerned with the labor intensity of the treatment or the pain. They were focused on the peace of mind they had from being able to observe that there is an outlet for the malignancy, Johanna Brandt's "safety valve." Many patients who used salves had had some previous conventional treatment. These patients noted that the pain of the salves is nothing compared to either surgery or chemotherapy and that the side effects are far less than radiation. I was repeatedly told that while they understood the hesitancy herbalists

or even medical doctors might have in offering the salves to their patients, practitioners should not withhold the salve on the basis of its potential for causing itching and burning.

Most patients did state that wider understanding of the escharotics would greatly facilitate their use since questions arise that cannot be answered by those inexperienced in the use of this method of cancer treatment. This book will, of course, fill a void that has been in existence for centuries; but I must go on record stating that, like many of my predecessors, I regard this treatment as a method of surgery, not an alternative to surgery but a unique method of surgery. As such, I also believe that except for the simplest and most superficial tumors, the treatment does require the assistance of experts.

CHAPTER 14

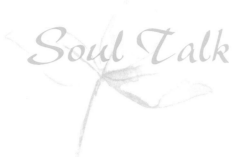

Soul Talk

As I come to the end of a labor that has consumed most of the prime of my life, I am feeling reflective and self-analytical. I saw my first cancer patient in 1972. At that time, I was clairvoyant and had the ability to see not only the aura but also the insides of the body by use of a sort of x-ray vision that occurred spontaneously. My knowledge of health and healing arose first from these insights and only later from "study." I valued the gifts greatly, but my destiny entailed surrender of some of my mystical proclivities in order to approach "reality" a little more directly. It has now been twenty-seven years since I first began brooding on treatment options for severely ill persons.

The material in this book is offered as one body of knowledge, probably the most practical presentation of information of my career. Its worth depends on the role the treatment strategies play for those people who most need help or who, as professionals, are seeking a more humane and natural option to current cancer treatments.

As I review and assess what I have put into the book, I am, on the one hand satisfied with what I have written. At minimum, I have demystified a treatment that has enjoyed hundreds of years of patient and professional acceptance. At maximum, I have earned the right to prod those with proper facilities and training to take a harder look at where this treatment belongs in the health care world— and more importantly, I have discussed a reasonable alternative, one I would myself use if "the shoe were on the other foot."

PRECIOUS GIFTS

Thus, if my enthusiasm for the salves—and their accompanying tonics—has been couched in various cautious statements, it has to be understood that it is not because of the remedies but rather the enormity of my own view of the healing process—and my measured assessment of how much patients can reasonably expect to achieve when directing their own healing. The desire to be in control, often given as a reason for using the salves, is laudable but fraught with risks, mainly of the very unpredictable reactions that attend use of bloodroot products.

NATURE

My uncle was an oceanographer who wrote ponderous books on marine biology and, at the end of his life, a little treasury of private thoughts. Of the many pearls in that tiny book was a sentence I have never been able to forget: "If you wish to understand Nature, do not disturb Her."

I do not know that we are today "observing Nature" in any meaningful way. We see Her as something to be manipulated. We wish to deprive Her of Her secrets but not offer our gratitude and reverence in exchange. Where phytopharmaceuticals are concerned, we "divide and conquer:" we break plants into their constituents and try to determine which parts are active in the fight against this or that disease. Then, we try to profit by the "discovery" and synthesize the chemical components that we perceive as important, casting away that which we do not understand or that we regard as non-important.

In my studies of Eastern methods of healing, I learned that Tibetans believe that the component of the herbs that is healing is the light. In fact, all nourishment is light. Plants transform light into foods that we can consume. In so doing, they perform a divine service and offer us a method of anchoring more

Heaven on Earth. In my mind, this is how deep and lasting healing will occur.

Additionally, though we may recognize the power of a particular chemical to destroy malignancy or retard mitogenic activity, the other constituents of herbs may protect organs from damage while the cytotoxins are carrying out their functions. This is what makes herbal medicine holistic. If we can be relatively certain that the body is being healed at the same time that the cancer is being eradicated, we can rest in the graciousness of Nature and allow Her to do what She does best: maintain balance.

I have an enormous respect for and love of herbs. Botanical remedies appeal to me on the basis of their willing service to life as well as their capacity to heal without harming. Perhaps I am lacking stoicism; but I am also unconvinced that those who have made sacrifices in the name of cure have done so wisely.

My own Path has carried me through many severe health challenges. As a child, my parents dragged me to doctors they regarded as hugely skilled whom I perceived mainly as arrogant or massively limited. It was only when I discovered Ayurveda and herbs that I found medicines that appealed to common sense and my personal desire to avoid repugnant substances.

For those who have not delved into these subjects to the same extent as I have, it may not be clear how dependent Western medicine is on diagnosis and how treatment stems from assumptions directly related to the diagnosis. On balance, this view of medicine is a bit more static than true life—which is always changing.

For example, Kirlian photographs of cancer cells suggest that they change dramatically in response to toncs, sounds produced by tuning forks. Clairvoyants also tend to see cancer in a very fluidic way, perhaps accounting (at least partially) for the discrepancies in diagnosis that are so tormenting to those whose futures depend so much on the diagnoses.

Eastern medicine is energetic and perhaps as dynamic as Western medicine is focused on frozen moments in time. By this, I mean that a tissue sample that has been fixed is very different from a living one and a computer print out of a laboratory test is vastly different from a pulse. Moreover, there is much more to a pulse than its rate. All the systems of medicine from Asia have sophisticated methods of determining the state of every organ, the circulatory and eliminatory systems, nerves, and so forth by reference to the pulses and presenting symptoms. In these systems, each patient is unique and the causes underlying the symptoms can be deduced by the pulse and shall we say "texture of the patient."

For instance, fear may exhibit as a rapid and quite jumpy pulse. According to Jones, worry undermines "nerve power." Ayurvedic practitioners would agree; moreover, they would see that the stress of the anxiety would wear down the patient, sometimes to the extent that curative measures would be ineffective. It is thus crucial that the terror of treatment is banished so that healing can begin. There can be fear stemming from the realization that one has cancer, fear of the horror of the prescribed treatments, fear of what is not understood about the treatments, fear of the unknown, and so on and so forth. Personally, I see that these weakening influences can relate as much to allopathic treatments that are maiming and rife with side effects—but ostensibly reliable—as to more natural strategies that are perhaps less harmful but, in some instances, less understood and therefore less trusted.

It comes down to choices. It is for this reason that I urge upon each patient the need for a quick education. I have seen patients become so absorbed in researching their options that they fail to realize that they are not actually in treatment. It is for this reason that I advocated on what is called the "disclaimer page" a limited commitment to investigating options. Set aside a reasonable length of time for asking questions and then make a decision. In ten to twenty days, most patients can polish off a few books, such as those mentioned on page 213, and come to some realistic evaluations of what strategies seem relevant and acceptable in one's particular circumstances.

Thus, whereas I am keenly devoted to herbs and the more psychotherapeutic and spiritual aspects of healing, others may be so uncomfortable with these approaches that they opt for something that has more objective standards of assessment. In my opinion, the treatment must appeal to the whole person or parts of the person will reject the treatment. Therefore, just as Morrnah Simeona explained to me that the subconscious rejects what does not feel good, so I feel the rational mind rejects what it does not understand. We are, however, so out of touch with ourselves that we do not always know what is in our best interests. In this unknowing, we are vulnerable to the influences of those who think they know; but the truth is no one knows what is right for another person. It is for reasons such as these that I have presented my understanding of botanic treatments in the way I have. I firmly believe that if the rationale of the treatment does not make you hear little bells sounding in your inner being that the bells are probably not ringing. Asking others whether or not they are ringing is like going to a priest or psychologist to ask if you are in love. If you do not know, maybe it is because you are not in love but merely trying to convince yourself you are.

The Cure For Cancer

So, here we are at the end of the main part of the book. It is important for you to know that I am an eternal seeker; I do not claim to have all the answers, merely to be truthful. I have personal experiences, particular insights, rather strong preferences in favor of certain approaches to healing, but I do not wish to impose these on anyone. My purpose has been to share, to pierce the veil of secrecy surrounding these treatments, to interpret what I have discovered within the limitations of my own personal knowledge, and to offer whatever hope I can based on what I have uncovered. I truly love herbs and have written more on them in the appendix that follows, including some charming stories from various healing tra-

ditions that differ significantly from the Western model.

I want to close by reiterating that the salves are dramatic; they upstage other treatments because people can actually see the process as it occurs. However, I would never suggest that the salves constitute a sufficient response to cancer. Together with the adjunctive herbal tonics, they constitute a reasonable physical strategy for handling the tumors and certain physiological imbalances; but, over the years, I have seen people so involved in the physical measures they are using to defeat cancer that they forget life, love, and divinity. Hildegard emphasized the role of faith as well as "spiritual risk factors." In my estimation, patients often mistake belief for action. Our souls are here on earth for a purpose. If that purpose is not found and lived, the soul becomes discouraged and withdraws. This is the real cause of death. I have often told patients that cancer never kills anyone: the soul creates life and the soul takes it away.

I am a passionate person. My soul is on fire and can often soar, but when I come down to Earth, I am often overwhelmed with tears. I would urge each person facing cancer to seek Divine guidance. I would also urge living the Truth one finds—both in one's medical choices and personal life. Visualize, prioritize, harmonize, actualize, and realize your Dreams. Be loving, keep the Faith, and treat your body and your life as a precious gift from God.

More I cannot say except to part with my personal blessings for your health and healing.

Appendices

APPENDIX A

Anticancer Herbs

ANY HERBS have been used in cancer treatment. Jim Duke, formerly of the United States Department of Agriculture (USDA), noted that the National Cancer Institute has screened 35,000 herbs and found 3000 of these to have some "activity against cancer." Dr. Jonathan Hartwell tracked 5000 years of ethnopharmacological history. His findings were published in eleven installments in *Lloydia* between 1967 and 1971. Hartwell reported on medicinal uses of plants from ancient China, Egypt, Greece, and Rome. He surveyed Islamic, European, Native American, and modern sources. He, too, cited references to about 3000 herbs used in a variety of ways, internally and externally, for cancer treatment.

Hartwell's work on cancer herbs began with studies on podophyllin, a resin isolated from the rhizomes of *Podophyllum peltatum*, the may apple. This is the plant used by the Penobscot Indians for the treatment of cancer. In a routine study of the literature on this plant, Hartwell learned that it had been used

by physicians in Mississippi and Louisiana in the nineteenth century. This clued Hartwell in to the fact that folklore could be a resource for information on cancer treatment, something the Harvard trained chemist had not considered before identifying the chemical agents in the may apple that were responsible for its anticancer activity (in mice). May apple is not covered in this book. Though most of my sources on Native American medicine cited may apple as a treatment for cancer, none referred to its use in escharotics.

I am acutely aware that professional botanists and medical herbalists have at their disposal the same references available to me. This section is not therefore intended to be a complete discussion of anticancer herbs. Rather, my objective has been to present enough information on a few of the key herbs used in escharotic formulae and their adjunctive healing salves and tonics to persuade skeptics as to the medical basis of a few older traditions. It is also my hope that the tidbits, for this is all they are, of information here presented will help patients to develop an appreciation of the gifts Nature offers the inhabitants of this diverse Planet. If the forging of the important body-mind connection is in any way assisted by my efforts, I will be content. Thus, while highly unorthodox, I begin with Hildegard of Bingen's herbs, but not from the insights of St. Hildegard herself, because I found some absolutely delightful stories of Native American origin that related to the same herbs.

My purpose has not been to catalogue what science has proved. What happens to a transplanted tumor has never seemed the same to me as what happens when a malignancy occurs spontaneously. I am therefore more inclined to credit clinical experiences, however anecdotal, than what happens in laboratories.

This said, truth must be the same no matter how it is discovered. Thus, whether the healing gifts of a plant are revealed to the eyes of a mystic or the mind of a scientist, the facts remain essentially the same. I have always felt that intuition and intellect need to merge. If the perceptions and analyses are clear, the findings will support each other—whereas biases, of whatever degree of certitude, merely obscure both the observations and the conclusions based on the data. The possibilities that open when the gaps in methodology are bridged are endless. A case in point is the well-reported ethnobotanical uses of the Madagascar periwinkle, a plant containing the alkaloid vincristine. This plant has cytostatic actions that work much like a drug; and its chemical derivatives have been used to make vincristine and vinblastine, chemotherapeutic drugs.

Given the number of plants with anti-cancer properties, it is a pity that so few have been put to medical use. It may also be lamented that when the medicinal value of plants is recognized, the profit motive dictates that synthetic forms of the pharmacologically active constituents be developed.

Some plants are potent and have side effects similar to pharmaceutical drugs. For example, use of a strong alkaloid that inhibits mitosis and cell growth can be debilitating when used for long periods of time. Some herbs are quite poisonous, even deadly. Yet, the rationale that governs use of dangerous drugs in medicine is often applied to medical herbalism, and such plants are therefore sometimes used on a restricted basis for short periods of time.

THE DISMAL PAST

In the course of researching this book, there have been some disappointments. First was the secrecy surrounding the exact recipes and protocols used by those who claimed to be successfully treating cancer. Next was centuries of relentless persecution of several of history's most prominent practitioners. Hoxsey's troubles with the law were nothing new but more a dismal continuum dating as far back as the Inquisition. Lastly was the fact that the major interest in botanical cures for cancer has not arisen within the medical establishment, but rather within the environmental community. Despite countless studies indicating that thousands of herbs may offer people suffering from cancer more promise than conventional protocols, concern for deforestation has been the main force behind ethnobotanical research. The eradication of herbs vitally needed by mankind has become an environmental instead of medical issue. The realization that humanitarian considerations have not prevailed over industrial motives in medicine and pharmacology has been a blow to my personal idealism.

Thousands of well-informed patients are perhaps needed to make a difference in this bleak picture. A cancer patient once asked me why AIDS patients demonstrate and cancer patients go like lambs to the slaughter. Though idiosyncrasies of temperament may account for some of the behavioral differences, I think entrenchment and indoctrination are the main factors behind the current state of affairs in cancer treatment. I was taught to have respect for scientists and made to believe that their thinking was not fettered by either convention or the desire for a particular outcome. Medical academia is today far from this standard, and this situation can only work to the advantage of industry at the expense of patients.

Modern Herbalism

For years, professional herbalists have been warned to stay away from cancer. Medical herbalists may treat gallstones and candida albicans but not cancer. Patients need to understand that years of training go into becoming proficient in any profession. Healing is not an exception to this rule; it requires an extensive education. Medical doctors study a certain curriculum and acquire considerable expertise in the intricacies of their field. Chiropractors, acupuncturists, naturopaths and medical herbalists, and others also have expertise, but they have been "restrained from trade" where cancer is concerned. There is no sound basis for awarding this monopoly to allopathic medicine. If the war on cancer were being won, there might be some grounds for arguing the superiority of conventional medicine over holistic medicine. However, the war is not being won; and countless people have suffered in the name of science. An additional consequence of years of monopoly is that alternative medicine does not have either the funding or current studies needed to defend its tenets. My investigation of escharotics has been hampered by lack of data, but my frustrations have been nothing compared to those of patients earnestly trying to become well.

As it stands today, if a lay person were to pick up a few herb books in search of something on cancer, likely as not the information would be quite vague and perhaps also couched in oblique but safe references to some historic use of a particular herb by some ethnic group or other. Instructions for use of the herb would probably be omitted. The patient would not therefore know whether to use the leaves, flowers, roots, bark, or seeds or whether to use the fresh or dry or tinctured herbs singly or in combination with other herbs. This is exactly what has happened with the "bloodroot story" in recent years. Resourceful patients track down some bloodroot and then do not know which part of the plant to use, whether to take it internally or externally, what dosage to use, how to prepare the poultices or pastes, how to bandage, how to interpret what is happening at the treatment site, how long to continue, etc. Though this book addresses some of the questions surrounding use of bloodroot, patients are entitled to access to whatever additional information they might need to improve their health. Moreover, they should be able to obtain preparations as well as guidance in their use from a qualified medical herbalist without fear of reprisal. Moreover, these services and treatments should be covered by insurance! At present, we are far from this ideal.

CLARIFICATION

Some remedies used in cancer treatment have been debunked due to failure to prove that an individual herb has specific antitumoral properties. For the most part, this should not be a cause of concern. The fact that an herb was used for people with cancer does not necessarily mean that the herb has anticancer action. It may have been used to decongest the liver or bowels, relieve lymphatic stagnation, promote metabolism or perspiration, stimulate circulation, raise immunity, or prevent infection. Or, it could be included in a formula because of its synergy with other herbs or its capacity to protect internal organs from dam-

age while treatment of the more life-threatening condition is necessary.

It is beyond the scope of this book to interpret the actions of the many herbs used in cancer treatment. I am simply warning that the absence of a demonstrable antitumoral effect on the part of a specific herb does not lead ipso facto to a conclusion that a person with cancer is wasting his time and money by taking the formula. While there are reasons for performing tests, trials are seldom performed on real people with cancer. For the most part, research findings are based on the actions of a single herb or constituent of that herb, not the action of the formula in which the herb is but one ingredient. There is little in the nature of such tests that could possibly indicate whether or not a person might benefit by use of the remedy.

In fact, use of laxative, stimulating, regenerative and many other types of herbs may not only promote well being but also assist overall healing. However, whether or not an herb is beneficial will depend on its quality, its proper use, and the patient's ability to assimilate it. Some people who ingest tablets or capsules eliminate them whole; the medicine passes through the entire gastrointestinal system without being absorbed, and it is, of course, useless to the patient if not assimilated. There is also such a thing as being overly aggressive, especially with cancer treatment. In excess, what promises much may actually destroy. Some persons were able to eliminate cancer entirely only to die of liver failure. Thus, the difference between killing cancer and healing the patient may be quite significant—and explain the need for a truly holistic approach to treatment.

Violets

I recently bought a very sweet book called *Song of the Seven Herbs* by Walking Night Bear (Dr. Henryk Binder). It is based on Native American folklore. I was intrigued by the fact that Hildegard's two main cancer remedies, violets and yarrow, were among the seven herbs whose "tales" were related in the book. What follows is my attempt to paraphrase and abbreviate the stories.

The Little People used to live in caves on a great mountain named Tomuni. They spent their time helping those who were sick. The walls of the caves were made of crystals that imparted strength and wisdom to the Little People. In one corner, there was a small dark amethyst who listened to stories told by the Mountain Spirit while the Little People gathered around the fire at night. As the Little Amethyst listened to the stories, he longed to see the earth from the outside of the cave and to help those who were sick. After many, many years, joy turned to sadness when the story of people with lumps on their bodies reached the Little People. They called Tomuni and told him that the lumps poisoned the blood and the spirit and that many die of this condition. The Little People could find no herbs to help the people who were sick because of these lumps.

Tomuni said that he had been thinking of this problem but had not found a solution.

Little Amethyst heard this and began praying to the Great Spirit and offered himself to help. The Creator then appeared as a light in the cave and stood before Little Amethyst saying that for some time He had been aware of the noble wish in Little Amethyst's heart to help the people who are sick. He told Little Amethyst that he would suffer greatly if he left the safety of the cave. Despite this warning, Little Amethyst was fervent in his wish to help. So, the Creator lifted Little Amethyst from the rock where he had so long resided and listened to the fireside stories. He was then transformed into a little green plant with the shape of a heart. The Creator carried him from the cave, down the mountain, and into a wooded area, and there He planted Little Amethyst. With the help of Mother Earth, Little Amethyst soon had many children. Then, another miracle happened: a beautiful flower blossomed. It was the same color as Little Amethyst had once been as a crystal in the cave.

The Little People told the medicine man of Little Amethyst. The medicine man was very happy and said that since Little Amethyst was no longer a crystal, he needed a new name. He looked to the sky. The sun had just set. The medicine man spoke, "From now on, your name shall be Violet, the color of the amethyst and the sky at sunset." The plant was very happy because he now had a beautiful name and the means to make people with lumps well. However, the Creator was right: life for the plant and its children was very hard. It was difficult to bear the hot sun so it learned to hide its flowers inside its leaves—and many did not realize that they tromped on the flowers when they walked. Little Violet was, however, so full of love that he bore no grudge for the pain this caused him. Even today, Little Violet loves to listen to stories told by good people who sit by the fire.[83]

As this Native American story suggested, violets have heart-shaped leaves and deep blue to purple flowers. They are Venus ruled and are used to cool excess heat anywhere in the body. Homer told of how Athenians used violets to "moderate anger." Culpeper stated the flowers of white violets dissolve swellings.

Dorothy Hall[84] writes metaphysically of violets. First, she notes that they have a curious way of "walking" to another part of the garden. Plant them one place, find them the next season in another, the original plants having withered. She also discusses their chameleon-like odor. Violets are wonderfully fragrant, but they absorb other odors and lose their own aroma. She states that violets even absorb the odor of death itself. While attempting to describe violets in a lecture, she observed the similarities between the lymphatic system and violets and noted that violets restore lymph flow.

Violet flowers are expectorants and the roots are emetic. In the 1930s, violets were used after surgery to prevent the development of secondary tumors. They were also used to treat breast and lung cancer. Today, violet leaf tincture is used for lymphatic stasis, blood-component changes, and spleen enlargement. The leaves are antiseptic and are used internally and externally for the treatment of malignancies. Crushed violet leaves can be applied to external lesions in lieu of an antiseptic. They can also be used to treat severe eczema in children. Violets are antitumoral. Contemporary British medical herbalists use the flowers and leaves to treat breast and stomach cancer. Strong infusions are taken every two to three hours. Add two ounces of leaves to one pint of boiling water. Let the brew stand overnight, strain, and drink two fluid ounces at a time.

Yarrow

Hildegard of Bingen prescribed yarrow to prevent metastasis. She also advised taking it as protection before surgery and for some time afterwards until healed. Doctors in Europe who work with "Hildegard Medicine" state that yarrow is also protective against the harmful side effects of radiation.[85]

The yarrow story in *Song of the Seven Herbs* relates that there were once people who lived in such peace and reverence that an envious man who lived near the Peyote peoples poisoned their water. The people and the animals, including the elderly medicine man, became very sick. The medicine man sent his grandson, Climbing Bear, to fetch some yarrow from the mountains. Climbing Bear did not reach the place where yarrow grew until nightfall. Climbing Bear called to the spirits for help, telling them that he needed light to see in the dark so he could find what his people needed before they perished. As he looked up, he saw pieces of stars breaking off and falling like snow. They landed right on the yarrow. Climbing Bear collected as much of the herb as was needed and used his last strength to return to his people. His grandfather made a tea for all the people and animals, and everyone was soon again healthy. Even now, if you go out at night, you can find the yarrow because the little stars are still shining.

The botanical name of yarrow is *Achillea millefolium*. The plant was named for Achilles, the Trojan war hero with the Achilles heel who healed his wounded soldiers with a genus of yarrow. Dioscorides, physician for the Roman Army, rubbed the crushed plant on wounds. When I first began studying herbs, I read that the word yarrow came from *guerra* or war. For many years I was prejudiced against the plant because I associated it with war rather than healing. In fact, the English name comes from the Anglo-Saxon *gearuwe* meaning "healer," not "war." Alternate names for yarrow include "soldier's woundwort," the name used during the Civil War, and "herba militaris." Like the Romans, Ute warriors (from Utah) crushed the herb and applied it to minor wounds.

Yarrow is a perennial herb belonging to the thistle family. It grows nearly everywhere. Many regard the plant as a weed, but I planted mine to hold the soil on a piece of land sloping towards my house. Several patients consulting me believed yarrow to be poisonous so early one morning I invited them to watch wild rabbits having breakfast. One particularly beautiful evening, I was admiring the elegant, feathery leaves of the yarrow. The next morning, I awakened to find that the rabbits had eaten those same delicious leaves. The rabbits living near my house keep my plants well champed, but only the medicinal plants. They do not eat the showier ones that are within a foot or so of the medicinal ones.

In earlier times, yarrow was used in divination, this from Europe all the way to China where the sticks are thrown to determine the hexagrams of the I Ching. Astrologers gave Venus rulership over yarrow and used chants together with yarrow to invoke romance into life.

Maude Grieve wrote that Highlanders make an ointment from yarrow that they apply to wounds. She also says that people in the Orkneys use it to dispel melancholy. This is, of course, the humor historically associated with the cancer temperament. Norwegians chew the leaves to cure toothaches. In Sweden, it is called "field hop" and is used in beer. Linnaeus (1707–1778) felt that yarrow was more intoxicating than hops. Yarrow is regarded by some as a sedative or even as a mildly hypnotic herb because of the presence of small amounts of thujone.

The leaves, stems, and flowers of yarrow are gathered in August, dried, powdered, and made into teas, one-half to one ounce of the herb to one pint of water. The tea should be steeped for at least five minutes. For fevers, drink a small glass of this tea every few hours. The tea helps to open the pores and purify the blood.

The aromatic properties of yarrow are strongest in the flowers and the astringency, which is used to staunch the flow of blood, in the leaves. The Greeks regarded the herb, also known as "nosebleed," as a styptic and vulnerary. It contains two substances, achilletin and achilleine, which promote blood clotting following injury. Culpeper said to boil a decoction with white wine to control fluids. This drink relaxes the blood vessels and improves circulation. Eclectics used the herb for incontinence, hemorrhage, and menstrual cramps.

As noted, Native Americans used the herb to treat wounds. More recent use is similar to that of the Eclectics: the herb has been used to stop internal bleeding and involuntary urination; but today, yarrow is primarily valued for its use in colds and influenza. Yarrow is also a circulatory aid, and it is valuable in regulating the menstrual cycle and flow and well as spasm (cramps). The flowers are rich in substances that reduce allergic reactions and control hay fever. The flowers must be steamed to release these volatile oils. The essential oil is anti-inflammatory and pain relieving. Yarrow contains cineol, a natural antiseptic. Yarrow may also be a rather potent heart remedy.

Despite its long history of medicinal usage, yarrow is somewhat poorly researched. Experiments conducted on patients suggest that it stimulates gastric secretions and improves digestion. Animal studies show that the extract is calming and that it reduces inflammation. Test tube studies demonstrate antibiotic effects. Two studies conducted on animals showed that yarrow protects the liver from toxic chemical damage. An Indian study proved yarrow useful in treating hepatitis. Since other members of the thistle family are among the most important herbs used for liver regeneration, these findings should not sur-prise herbalists. What is important is the relationship between these modern findings and historic uses such as Hildegard and the Peyote people described.

Bloodroot

Bloodroot is indigenous to North America. It grows in the East from Canada to the Carolinas and sometimes as far south as Florida. Its botanical name is *Sanguinaria canadensis*. When the root is cut, it appears to bleed. Native Americans used this red exudation as a dye for decorating the body as well as textiles. Bloodroot is thus sometimes known as red puccoon or Indian paint. The history of bloodroot is as colorful as the dye made from it.

Bloodroot flowers very early in the spring, March or April. The flowers are usually white with seven to fourteen petals, but they are sometimes tinged with rose or purple. They close in the shade and at night. It is the root that is most often used in medicine. The roots are small, finger thickness, and only 2–3 inches in length.

The medicinal uses of bloodroot were learned from Native Americans in the Lake Superior region. The roots are prepared into pastes and ointments, washes, and tinctures, and used either singly or in combination with other herbs. Indians also pulverized the roots to use as a snuff for cases of nasal polyps.

Bloodroot is considered highly effective against most skin conditions, everything from ringworm to warts, fungoid tumors, and vene-real infections. For athlete's foot, eczema, rashes, and fungal infections, washes may be preferred to the salve. The famous "black salve" or "Compound X," known from the Great Lakes to the West Coast and all the way south to Tierra del Fuego, is a paste made with bloodroot and a number of other herbs or flour and water plus zinc chloride. It is this preparation that is used in the treatment of warts and tumors. Bloodroot is effective against gangrene infection as well. It is also used in a number of dental preparations for treatment of gingivitis and plaque and can be found as an ingredient in some brands of toothpaste.

Research has established that bloodroot has a remarkable ability to remove mucus. For this purpose, it may be taken internally in small doses; but, when taken internally, it should never be used in large doses or for a prolonged period. Perhaps, its nasty taste is Nature's way of warning against overuse internally.

Bloodroot is both bitter and pungent. Initially, bloodroot warms and stimulates, but then its cooling properties overcome the heating ones so that bloodroot can be used to reduce fever and inflammation. The primary alkaloid in bloodroot, sanguinarine, has been determined to be an potent anticancer agent. In experiments on mice, sanguinarine had a necrotizing effect both carcinomas and sarcomas.

Externally, bloodroot is prized for its ability to clear up infections and stimulate the growth of healthy tissue. So far as can be determined, bloodroot is the most common herb used in escharotic treatments. Historically, it was usually combined with other herbs, such as mandrake, poke root, galangal, goldenseal, yellow dock, blue flag, and roasted red onions. Some tribes added jimson seeds, *Datura stramonium*, to bloodroot to reduce pain. The Zuñi of New Mexico have a wonderful story about the *a'neglakya* plant, named for a boy who lived in the interior of the earth. The powdered root is a narcotic, but externally, it is applied to wounds of all type. The Cherokee also used *datura* with puccoon, either bloodroot or perhaps goldenseal.

In the last century, bloodroot was often mixed with Kali tartaricum (cream of tartar) or zinc chloride. Today, it is combined with other herbs with known antitumor effects: burdock, sheep's sorrel, and red clover as well as the traditional galangal and zinc chloride. Some producers have added turmeric and/or DMSO or MSM to the traditional recipes.

Galangal

Galangal is a member of the ginger family. It was first introduced into Europe by Arab physicians in the 9th century. Hildegard of Bingen called it the "spice of life," given by God to ward off ill health. It is a major spice in Thai cooking and has a wonderful, exotic taste that adds much delight to Thai food. It is native to southern China and Southeast Asia. The root is used in medicines, either fresh or dried. In general, it is considered to be a stomachic and a useful treatment and preventative for motion sickness.

Research in China showed that a decoction of galangal had antibacterial action. Studies published in 1988 showed it to be effective against candida albicans. It is a common ingredient in escharotic pastes, the one that accounts for the somewhat exciting smell of the "black salves."

Goldenseal

Goldenseal grows naturally in the Carolinas and Appalachias north to Ontario. Its botanical name, *Hydrastis canadensis*, suggests its affinity for the north. Goldenseal has a small white to rose colored flower and a single inedible fruit. It grows from eight to twenty inches in height and has three to five green lobed leaves. Its root is gnarly and very bitter, indication of the presence of an alkaloid—one with truly extraordinary medicinal properties.

Though the Cherokee are most often credited with teaching the early colonists the use of goldenseal, many other tribes were conversant with the medicinal uses of goldenseal: the Blackfoot, Crow, Iroquois, and Seminole. Goldenseal is sometimes called yellow root or yellow puccoon. Indians used the root as a yellow dye or mixed it with indigo to create a green color.

The Cherokee used goldenseal for a variety of conditions: bleeding, disinfection, congestion, fevers, heart problems, digestive disorders, and liver ailments. The root mixed with bear fat was used as an insect repellent and lotion for wounds, ulcers, and sores. Indians also chewed the root to cure mouth sores. Benjamin Smith Barton wrote in 1798, "I am informed that the Cherokee cure cancer with a plant which is thought to be the *Hydrastis canadensis*." Lewis and Clark wrote that Indians used the root to cure sore eyes. As noted earlier in this book, goldenseal was at one time so much in demand that it nearly became extinct. Today, it is seldom found in the wild but is cultivated commercially albeit with some difficulty. It likes shade and fertile, moist soil near rivers.

Goldenseal was introduced to Europe in 1760 and obtained official recognition as a result of a medical paper published in 1798. Samuel Thomson called it goldenseal in an 1833 publication. The Eclectics held goldenseal in very high esteem. They described the root as a styptic with hemostatic and healing properties. It will also be recalled that Dr. John Pattison preferred goldenseal to bloodroot for use in his enucleating paste. He not only used goldenseal in his paste but also administered tinctures and homeopathic remedies made from the root as additional constitutional treatments for cancer. He was convinced that goldenseal has a specific action on malignancy that was superior to that of other escharotic preparations in his day (1866).

Goldenseal is a bitter tonic, one which stimulates the secretion of bile and bilirubin. It tones the liver and gall bladder. The two active alkaloids, hydrastine and berberine, have been isolated and tested. They have been discussed in journals in this century as ideal for treating mucous surfaces. Goldenseal is considered an official pharmaceutical in eleven countries. Japanese studies indicate that goldenseal has extremely potent antibacterial activity. Dr. Daniel B. Mowrey states that goldenseal increases T-cell activity and other immunological functions. He warns that prolonged use can result in overproduction of leucocytes since goldenseal does not discriminate between deficiency and excess, it merely stimulates.[86] Since echinacea does make the distinction, many herbalists recommend using goldenseal in conjunction with echinacea. Berberine is a constituent of several other herbs, such as barberry and Oregon grape root, herbs that are used in internal tonics such as the famous trifolium compound of the Eclectics.

Berberine is extremely active against tumor cells; it destroys through increasing the activity of macrophages. It is even effective with brain tumors. According to Mowrey, the kill rate for berberine was 91% as compared to 43% for chemotherapeutic drugs. This study was done in vitro, but goldenseal does apparently have the ability to cross the blood-brain barrier. Berberine has been used in China to restore white blood cell counts after chemotherapy. It is highly protective against anemia. It is also helpful in increasing cardiac flow.

Berberine is an antibiotic, useful against serious infectious organisms such as E. coli, staphylococcosis, streptococcosis, chlymydia, salmonella, typhi, candida albicans, corynebacterium diphtheria, vibrio cholera, diplococcus pneumonia, and giardia. In laboratory tests, it was found to be more effective than chloramphenicol against certain bacteria.[87] Studies done in India show that it is also effective against cholera and amoebic infectious agents.

Marigold

Calendula officinalis is a very well known herb, native to Southern Europe, but it grows in temperate climates practically everywhere. Gardeners know that marigold is planted not merely for its decorative attributes but its capacity to ward off insects. What is not so well known is that marigold relieves the pain and swelling of bee and wasp stings.

The flowers of the marigold are harvested as they open in early summer. They are dried in the shade so as to prevent discoloration of the petals, which are then made into ointments or infusions to use on burns, eczema, fungal infections, and inflamed skin. Taken internally, calendula exhibits some of the same properties. It prevents suppuration and is used to treat ulcers and varicose veins. Calendula is antiseptic, antifungal, antibacterial, and antiviral. Marigold is used to detoxify and cleanse the liver and gall bladder. It has a mild estrogenic action and is used to relieve menstrual irregularities and discomfort. Pattison mixed a calendula ointment into his goldenseal enucleating paste. According to his description of this method, the goal was to keep the treatment site as calm as possible. Marigold may therefore have been used to reduce swelling and pain as well as to disinfect the treatment site.

Red Clover

Eclectic physicians and their successors in this century regarded red clover, *Trifolium pratense*, as a blood purifying herb. Red clover is quite high in iron as well as copper. It is the key herb in the traditional trifolium compound, an internal tonic similar to or identical with the famous Hoxsey *Elixirex,* Dr. John Christopher's black dogwood combination, Chief Sundance's anticancer elixir. Red clover grows nearly everywhere in the world and has hence been used as a common household remedy for centuries. Sometimes, red clover tea, combined with large amounts of garlic is used to defend against infection.

It is the blossoms that are used medicinally. They should be harvested in the morning as soon as the dew has evaporated. Then, they should be allowed to dry without exposure to direct, bright sun light.

Despite its popular domestic use, red clover has been difficult for herbalists to classify. It is traditionally considered to be Mercury ruled, is calming, and helps to soothe the nerves and improve the memory.

Red clover's action is rather slow; use therefore has to be continued for months. It is taken internally as a tea, tincture, or syrup. Externally, it can be used singly or in combination with other herbs as a poultice, liniment, or salve. One teaspoon of red clover blossoms to a cup of boiling water (pure water) makes a simple poultice, but red clover is more often made into salves or ointments. It is often used on skin cancers but it is most prized for its effectiveness with breast and ovarian cancers. Red clover can also be used in enemas and douches.

Used consistently, it helps to dissolve deposits, including malignancies. It reduces swelling and promotes urination. It aids tissue repair and relieves pain. The National Cancer Institute (NCI) has identified four antitumor compounds in red clover, including genistein.

Poke Root

Like bloodroot and goldenseal, poke is native to the Eastern part of the United States though its natural habitat extends somewhat further to the south than the red and yellow puccoons. It can sometimes be found in Minnesota and Texas. Species with properties similar to *Phytolacca americana* can be found in Mexico, South America, the West Indies, and Ethiopia. Millspaugh listed "cancer root" as one of the many names of poke.[88] Some of the other names by which poke root is known are pigeon berry, ink berry, American nightshade, and kermesberro, the name used by The Herb Finder. Its botanical name is *Phytolacca decandra*. According to herbal historians, poke root was one of the most valued herbs in the early American colonies. In the mid-eighteenth century, papers on its use were published, and the root was exported to Europe and even to the Black Sea area where it became known as *Fitalaka Americana.*

Poke grows wild in dry, waste soils. It has small greenish-white flowers that appear in July and August and dark purple berries that ripen later in the summer. In the South, the tender young shoots are used in salads as a substitute for asparagus, and the seedlings are eaten like spinach and other cooked greens; they may also be parboiled and used in tempura.

Since the active properties of the herb deteriorate rapidly with storage, most practitioners prefer to use the fresh green root soon after harvesting. Tinctures, cerates, and homeopathic remedies are also made from the root. Though somewhat less usual, the berries and occasionally even the leaves are used in decoctions. The fruit is also sometimes used medicinally (internally), and the dried berries have been used in plasters for cancer.

Though most often used externally, it is believed by some that internal use of poke will cut recovery time in half; but the root must be used sparingly when taken internally as it can cause vomiting. Its slightly warming properties make it a metabolic stimulant and ideal for overcoming stagnation and sluggishness of the bile or lymph. Many Eclectic physicians as well as Dr. John Christopher felt that poke was the herb of choice for inflammation, swelling, and cases of hardening of the glands, especially the thyroid, spleen, or liver. Due to its effects on catabolism, it has been used (in small doses) to promote deeper assimilation where there is severe malnourishment or emaciation. REPEAT: *great care should be taken when using this herb, since, in larger doses, poke root is an emetic, a rather slow acting but violent emetic.*

I brought some fresh poke root back from Georgia and gave it to my office manager who ran it through her juicer and put the pulp into a compost bucket on the floor of her kitchen. During the night, her big bouvier des Flanders got into the bucket. The sounds that came from this poor dog were dreadful. Maya survived just fine, but she had one awful night of vomiting.

Poke is a potent herb. It is used to kill plant viruses, parasites, and snails. It has also been employed as a spermicide. It is especially useful in treatments involving the skin, liver, glands, breasts, and bones. It can be used for mastitis as well as benign and malignant growths. Internally, it alleviates toxemia and constipation, reduces swelling, and promotes tissue regeneration. Poke root is the strongest known blood purifying or alterative herb. It can be used in the case of extreme poisoning. The tincture is used internally, in small quantities for breast cancer and externally as a wash for uterine cancer.

Dr. Eli G. Jones said that phytolacca is about 40% caustic potash. He recommended that the green root of phytolacca be used in all cases of breast cancer where the breast is hard and painful and of a purplish hue. He prescribed five drops of the tincture every three hours. When the breast is open, bleeds easily (and the blood is dark and decomposed in appearance), Jones instead recommended homeopathic Lachesis (6X), ten drops in half a glass of water, one teaspoon every hour. He also made a syrup with poke root, gentian, and dandelion that he gave to elderly patients.

Poke made into an ointment, mixed with tallow, can be used for swellings, mastitis, and cancer; crushed, it can be made into a poultice for suppurating wounds. The grated root is sometimes applied directly to suppurating wounds or to the skin where the purpose is to promote heat. Several herb books cite poke root as a treatment for breast cancer. Consequently, many women have made poultices of the fresh root and applied these directly to the skin. Accordingly to the reports provided me, this method of use is as painful as the most aggressive escharotic. Great fortitude is required to persevere with these treatments.

In research, poke root has demonstrated "significant enhancing activity" on the ability of macrophages to kill sarcomas and malignant fibroblasts.[89] It also stimulates interleukin production and mitogenic response. There is no question but that poke is an important medicinal plant; but whether used internally or externally, poke root is intense and should be used cautiously.

Chaparral

Though not controversial at all among Native American *curanderos,* a few writers dispute the healing benefits of another important anticancer botanical. Chaparral, popularly known as creosote bush or greasewood, is a desert bush that grows abundantly in California, Nevada, Arizona, and New Mexico. Its botanical name is *Larrea divaricata.* Alma R. Hutchens reported that chaparral is an Indian name referring to over one hundred different botanical plant types.[90]

The pharmacological history of chaparral is impressive. Many sources report a story of an elderly man who had had three operations for a melanoma. When it recurred, he refused a fourth operation and drank chaparral tea. The growth disappeared; and over the course of many months, he regained twenty-five pounds.

A local woman with ovarian cancer had been given six months to live by her surgeon. She took chaparral in capsule form, went back to her surgeon who, astonished to see her still alive, recommended a second look operation. No evidence of cancer was found during this procedure. When she stopped by to see me, she expressed disappointment that the surgeon failed to show an interest in chaparral. She fished around asking me what I thought; I said that I should be asking her for advice.

Yet another woman began use of chaparral after attending a Native American gathering. Her condition was much more compromised than the New Mexican just mentioned. She did not seem to respond to chaparral, at least not in the manner she was taking it. She eventually resorted to more surgery and made a good recovery.

Many years ago, a chiropractor with whom I was well acquainted used chaparral for many months. In addition to having cancer of the gall bladder, she had been bitten by a centipede. Doctors recommended amputating her arm. She refused and was completely healed of both conditions. She is still alive, approximately thirty years after her ordeal.

Native Americans placed the leaves and twigs of chaparral into a vessel and poured boiling water over them and let the brew stand overnight. They drank a small amount before meals and at bedtime. Heated mixtures of chaparral in combination with other herbs can be used as poultices and plasters. I was once told that Indians harvest chaparral with strict attention to the Moon, but these instructions have somehow slipped my memory; I therefore include this comment for consideration.

In the scientific community, attention has been focused on chaparral's active constituent, nordihydroguaiaretic acid (NDGA), found in the resinous coating of the plant's leaves and stems. Industrially, NDGA is used as an antioxidant in fats and oils. Laboratory studies conducted on rats showed that chaparral effectively prevented colon cancer in 9 out of 14 rats given a chemical carcinogen. In another study, done in India, it showed 83% effectiveness. Many studies have indicated similar protective properties as well as the capacity to inhibit cell proliferation and DNA synthesis. NDGA also exhibits antibacterial and antiviral activity. Research at NCI showed that chaparral is a "very active agent against cancer."[91]

One theory of chaparral's action is that it acts to convert fermentation processes that are out of balance. Dr. John Christopher conjectured that chaparral stimulated the growth of healthy cells in such a way that unhealthy cells died and were pushed out of the body. Dr. William Kelley theorized that chaparral chelates toxins out of the body, especially from the liver and pancreas. Other sources report that chaparral inhibits the electron transport system of tumors so that they are deprived of the energy they need to exist.

Chaparral contains gums and resins as well as significant amounts of protein. It is antiseptic and tonifying and can therefore be used to purify as well as to rebuild. It has been known to improve eyesight and hair growth and to reduce infections as well as tumors. It is particularly valued in cases of leukemia, but is widely used in many other forms of cancer as well.

The herb is highly regarded among Native Americans whose first response to discovery of cancer is often a quest for local sources of the herb. Though chaparral is nontoxic, the FDA has asked that it be taken off the market. Local people in my part of the country are not aware of the FDA's recommendation and continue to consume it in fairly heavy doses despite its rather awful taste and smell.

Burdock

It would appear that the first recorded reference in the West[92] to the use of burdock, *Arctium lappa*, for cancer treatment was by the twelfth century mystic Hildegard of Bingen. Since then, burdock has managed to remain controversial, so much so that it is not mentioned in some books on herbal medicine, or it is given credit only as a diuretic. Occasionally, burdock is even misidentified.

Burdock is native to Europe but grows everywhere in the world, mainly along roadsides. Burdock has purple flowers that look like thistles, but it is actually a member of the daisy family. It derives its name from the French *bourre,* and its burrs cling mercilessly to animal fur and clothing. Its stalks can be stripped and cooked in much the same way as asparagus, or they can also be eaten raw with salad dressing. Burdock is sometimes found in grain coffee, herbal caffeine-free coffee substitutes. In some cultures, it is eaten instead of potatoes in soups, in pancakes, and as cutlets. The taste and texture of burdock are distinctive and somewhat difficult to describe. Most herb sources state that the taste is somewhere between asparagus and celery; however, it is a bit tangy and has a bite. One of my staff thought that burdock resembles Jerusalem artichokes more than asparagus; I find it as Zen-like as buckwheat noodles and tofu! The texture of burdock is quite tough but less fibrous than celery and certain other plant foods.

It is the roots of the first year's growth that are used both as food and medicine. Harvesting generally takes place before the flowers open, usually about July or sometimes August. The roots are long and slender, about an inch thick and one to three feet in length. I planted some in my garden and found that my birds will eat the enormous leaves which are, however, very bitter. Unlike the leaves, the roots are mucilaginous and slightly sweeter; yet they have a strong hypoglycemic action and have been used to treat diabetes.

Burdock has a reputation for aiding uterine complaints. Burdock can be used in poultices to reduce swelling; it is a tumor resolvent. It can be used in teas, tinctures, and tablets. Laboratory studies have demonstrated its effectiveness in reducing tumors in animals. In both German (1967) and Japanese (1986) scientific studies, burdock exhibited significant antifungal and antibacterial properties. It is also a very fine blood purifier and can even be used in cases of poisoning by venomous insects and snakes. As a blood purifying tea, it is often combined with yellow dock and sarsaparilla or dandelion.

Turmeric

Turmeric, *Curcuma longa*, is my favorite herb, so much so that my students nicknamed me "Turmeric Doctor." Though curcumin was isolated in 1842 as the active constituent of turmeric, this fascinating spice has, until very recently, been much neglected by Western herbalists. Turmeric is a tropical plant related to ginger; it grows in Asia and the West Indies as well as Hawaii where it is known as *olena*. Turmeric is probably best known as the ingredient that imparts to curry its yellow color. As its color may suggest, turmeric is high in vitamin C. It also contains a significant amount of potassium. Though many herbs have an effect on carcinogenicity, turmeric is the only culinary spice to be considered in this section on herbs (galangal was mentioned mainly in reference to its external use in the escharotic pastes). As a seasoning, turmeric is primarily bitter and only secondarily astringent and pungent.

It is the root of turmeric that is used in both cooking and medicine. The root is boiled, dried, and then powdered. Clinical studies discussing the medicinal properties of turmeric are just beginning to be published. Preliminary findings, based on studies with mice, showed that turmeric reduced the number of tumors as well as their mutagenicity (tendency of cells to divide). This should come as no surprise to Eastern herbalists because turmeric is known to reduce fertility, i.e., to limit proliferation. In a Chinese study, turmeric was shown to be 100 percent effective in preventing pregnancy in female rats.

Turmeric also has a potent effect on fats and oils. As a digestive aid, turmeric stimulates the flow of bile and hence fat metabolism. It also protects DNA against oxidative injury.[93] Turmeric can be added to oils to prevent rancidity. Laboratory studies indicate that turmeric is a more powerful antioxidant than vitamins C and E. It is also a free radical scavenger or inhibitor of free radical reactions. Turmeric has been shown to protect the liver from damage, even damage caused by alcohol, drugs, prescription medicines, and carcinogens.

Earlier in this book, it was noted that turmeric can be used to arrest bleeding and reduce scar formation. Traditionally, turmeric was used both internally and externally to promote rapid healing and to reduce scar formation. To understand its action, it may be easiest to think of turmeric as preventing clumping, clotting, and coagulation so that wherever there is a tendency for tissue to thicken or adhere to other tissues, turmeric tends to break up this stickiness. When applied externally, it is an effective topical anti-inflammatory agent. In Hawaii, fresh turmeric root is used to treat fungal infections.

In animal studies, turmeric was toxic to cancer cells within thirty minutes. Clinically, turmeric has been found effective in inhibiting the growth of lymphomas, perhaps because of its emulsifying properties. In addition, it gives symptomatic relief (from itching and pain) when used externally on cancerous lesions. Turmeric has also been shown to reduce the odor of cancer (in 90 percent of cases). Since it is tasty and has no known harmful side effects, it can be used freely as a seasoning or medicine by anyone wanting to improve digestion and perhaps also reduce the risk of cancer.

CONCLUSION

Though it is not my purpose to site all the studies conducted on herbs, spices, and foods that might protect against cancer (there are thousands of such substances), I would like to report the results of a study of mice with cancer done in India. Many spices were shown to extend life. Of these, black pepper, asafoetida, pippali, and garlic were the most significant. As a preventative against exposure to carcinogens, even more spices were found effective. This makes perfect sense to me since stagnation of energy may play a part in the development of cancer; and spices tend to be stimulating and hence to relieve congestion. South Indians, who are renown for their consumption of spices, have one of the world's lowest incidences of colon cancer.

Westerners who are not used to spices should begin with small amounts and increase the pungency of their meals little by little as they become accustomed to the taste. For those new to Eastern cuisine, I would suggest eating in Thai and Indian restaurants in order to become familiar with the tastes of the various dishes. Then, one can begin cooking at home with more spices.

APPENDIX B

Formulae

THE RECIPES AND FORMULAE included in this appendix represent my best effort to catalogue the current status of my investigations of escharotic treatments and their accompanying elixirs. Without exception, I have included all the details known to me. In some cases, this means that only the ingredients are listed. When the proportions were available, the information has been included. In only a few instances were the methods of preparation divulged. Again, when the instructions were provided, they have been reported in full. Since this has been an ongoing process for me, each edition has encompassed a fuller perspective on the treatment methods, but the work is not complete—and no one is more aware of this than I.

Escharotics have been used by such a wide array of practitioners that the gamut of knowledge encompassed by these persons must perforce reflect the diversity of those associated with the method. At one end of the spectrum, we have the gifted seer St. Hildegard of Bingen, and at the other end physicians with vast clinical experience such as J. Weldon Fell, John Pattison, and Eli G. Jones. In addition, there are no doubt wholly unqualified but sincere individuals whose information is hearsay, incomplete, and perhaps even inaccurate. In other words, the individuals whose work has been covered include the mystically enlightened, erudite, experienced and perhaps also the gullible.

A careful analysis of the energetics and specific properties of the herbs in these formulae may reveal the clinical basis for the successes claimed for this method throughout history. For this reason, I have included the escharotic salves and pastes as well as whatever adjunctive tonics, teas, tinctures, and homeopathic remedies were cited in the published works of the persons whose work I have investigated. I have also included recipes from people who are today making the pastes. I am certain that the assembling of this much information in one place will catalyze herbalists to develop products of even greater benefit to patients.

I recognize the shortcomings of this section. It would be wonderful to know what the proportions of the ingredients are, what the correct botanical identification of boar's tusk root is, and exactly how each of these preparations was administered and with what level of success. It would also be useful to know whether bloodroot, for example, was used in a dried or powdered form or whether it is advisable to use the fresh root—and if so, exactly when the root should be harvested. My sense is that some of the answers to these questions can be inferred by the fact that Fell and Pattison worked in London. They, therefore, imported the herbs used in their practices. Some of my sources state that bloodroot paste has a virtually indefinite shelf life, at least ten years. Others said the paste should be refrigerated. With poke root, we can be a bit more certain. It should be used fresh or as a tincture or cerate. Both Jones and Christopher often used poke root after the escharotic, but they used it in a variety of forms.

I am emphasizing these points because so many patients have, over the years, contacted me saying that they had rounded up all the ingredients mentioned in this or that book and that they wished to know how to put them together. In many cases, it would appear that what they located was so old and dried out that the herbs had probably lost much of their potency. Most were surprised to learn that the pastes are readily available and that much of their trouble had therefore been unnecessary.

For those completely new to escharotics, I should note that the consistency of the pastes is "adjusted" when used. Many older references suggested adding flour or water "as necessary." Since zinc chloride is deliquescent, the pastes tend to change according to humidity (and temperature). When ready to use the paste, it will sometimes be found to be too sticky to spread properly or too runny to contain. In these cases, something needs to be done to achieve the right consistency. Though adding flour or water was the common practice in the last century, I have often proposed that pastes that are too thick be softened a bit with a cerate. For this purpose, calendula may be the first choice, but preliminary trials with poke, lomatium, violet, and garlic have also been encouraging. When the paste is too thin, the usual recommendation has either been to add flour or more of the powdered herbs, in the same proportion as the original formula. However, adding goldenseal and/or turmeric powder works extremely well and tends to make for a "quieter," less inflamed treatment site. Since goldenseal is mucilaginous and turmeric is "crumbly," this strategy requires more attention to the final consistency.

My personal opinion is that the Pattison methodology is both easier on the patient and safer. It was based on the premise that the more trauma to the site can be reduced, the lower the risk of metastasis. For this reason, I am certain that, unless the tumor is very fast growing, the stronger alkaloids and lower concentrations of zinc chloride are superior. This said, it must be admitted that trials to substantiate this matter have not been performed.

Elixirs and Teas

The importance of the adjunctive tonics and teas cannot be over emphasized. Most practitioners using escharotics believed that the escharotics constituted a method of tumor removal that is less harmful than surgery. Only for this reason did they employ the method. For those who used them, the internal elixirs were nearly always regarded as more important than the escharotics. With many practitioners, herbal teas and powders were used to strengthen the particular systems of the body that were ravaged by disease or that may have contributed to the disease in the first place. Several, such as Pattison and Christopher, were convinced that the formulae that supported the overall health of the organs affected by disease were as important as the specific antitumoral preparations. Nearly all believed that the decongesting tonics were crucial to health. Hildegard's duckweed elixir and the various *trifolium compounds* were primarily digestive and eliminatory aids that only secondarily addressed the cancerous state of tissue.

The deeper appreciation for the elixirs than for the escharotics may be partially explained by the fact that most exponents of the escharotic method believed that cancer is a systemic condition. In nearly all the cases studied, these elixirs were prepared as syrups. I mention this because there are today many "Hoxsey" or "red clover" preparations containing the same herbs as *Elixirex,* but they are provided in tincture or capsule form. While this may appear to be pharmacologically sound, it does not conform at all to historic practices.

Patients and practitioners alike may be challenged by the use of such syrups since so many authorities advise the complete elimination of sugars from the cancer diet. However, traditionally, there was strong support for sweetened medicinal aids. Some contended that due to the degenerative nature of cancer, sweetness is needed to promote deeper tissue regeneration. Others view the syrups as better carriers for the herbs. In any event, neither herbalists nor patients should feel safe in assuming that because the ingredients are the same, the preparations are equal. If our forebears had the skill that they seem from the records to have had, we might be wise to begin by approximating their methodology as nearly as possible.

Homeopathic Remedies

Next, while not myself sufficiently conversant with homeopathy to comment extensively on the subject, I feel it necessary to report that Pattison and Jones relied quite heavily on the power of homeopathic remedies to affect the deeper constitutional patterns that they felt are not as easily impacted by the herbs. Since many are today as interested in homeopathy as in the time of Hahnemann, I have compiled, in chapters 7 and 8, a list of the remedies cited by Pattison and Jones, this despite the fact that I realize homeopaths have rather precise ways of determining which remedies to use and in what potencies.

ADJUNCTIVE TREATMENTS

Finally, though previously stated, it is no doubt good to repeat that though the phenomena attending the use of escharotics are often enough to persuade most patients and even some practitioners that this treatment is doing all the work, it is simply not sensible to neglect the adjunctive treatments that so many have found to be effective. Relieving stagnation of the lymphatic system, aiding digestion and elimination, detoxifying the liver and blood, enhancing immunity, destroying malignancy, regenerating organs, and promoting the growth of healthy new tissue are sound practices. In addition, there are diets and psychotherapeutic measures that can be tailored to the specific needs of individual patients. An adequate program probably requires the harmonization of many strategies.

The oldest herbal salve formula used on tumors known to the author comes from the mystic healer Hildegard of Bingen.[94]

Violet Salve

ANTITUMORAL SALVE

PARTS BY WEIGHT

3 parts	Violets
1 part	Olive oil
3 parts	Billy goat fat

Press the juice from the violets; strain through cheesecloth. Add the olive oil and billy goat fat. Boil in a clean pot and use as a salve on ulcerated tumors or any part of the body that hurts. This salve can also be used for "harmless" cysts in the connective tissue, lumps, precancerous growths, muscle sores, and headaches.

COMMENTS: according to Hildegard, the "viruses" will die when contacted by the salve.

PLEASE NOTE: German producers of this salve use violet flowers, not the whole plant, though both leaves and blossoms have anticancer properties.

Yarrow (achillea millefolium)

ANTI-METASTASIS BEVERAGE

First	Three pinches of powdered yarrow in fennel tea
Then	Three pinches of yarrow powder in warm wine

USE: to prevent metastases, Hildegard recommended using yarrow before surgery or after any internal injury. Use should be continued for at least eight days after surgery or injury or until completely healed. German physicians familiar with Hildegard's work suggest that yarrow also protects against radiation damage.

Duckweed Elixir

TO PREVENT "BAD JUICES" FROM FORMING IN THE STOMACH

Cinnamon	Sage
Ginger	Fennel
Rue	White pepper
Tormentil	Field mustard
Burdock	Wild bedstraw
Duckweed	

Filter these ingredients into duckweed (*Lemna minor*). Called honeywine elixir in *Hildegard's Medicine*.

DOSAGE: full sherry glass of the beverage is to be taken before meals and at bedtime for three months.

Anguillan

FOR PEOPLE WHO HAVE BEEN "INTERNALLY DAMAGED BY CANCER VIRUSES"

Eel gall	Long pepper
Basil	Ivory powder
Ginger	Powder from vulture's beak

PREPARATION: add these ingredients to the honeywine-vinegar extract.

COMMENTS: Hildegard said that the viruses in the body will get sick and die and cancer infested fatty tissue will regenerate if this remedy is taken. This action is attributed to the eel gall. Then, the vinegar dissolves the masses; the ivory causes them to dry up; and the vulture beak kills the rest.

PLEASE NOTE: vultures are a protected species. The beaks can only be harvested from vultures that have died as a result of accidents or natural causes. For this reason, homeopathic remedies have been developed from beaks acquired as a consequence of such deaths. German specialists recommend starting with D6, then D12, then D30, ten drops, six times a day in heart (warm) wine.[95]

USE: take for four to six weeks.

IMPORT: these two remedies are difficult to make. They are available in Germany and can be imported for personal use. See the author's web site for up-to-date ordering information:

http://www.cancersalves.com.

HISTORIC INDIAN REMEDIES

Poultices

Step One

1	Large red onion (roasted)
1 t.	Pocoon powder[96]

INSTRUCTIONS: make sure that the pocoon is finely powdered. Mix the powder well with the root of the onion. The plaster should be just large enough to cover the sore. Repeat every twelve hours until the body of the cancer assumes a deep purple or black color. Usually two plasters are enough. If the mass is really a cancer, this plaster will cause pain.[97]

Step Two

handful	Roasted young poke root
1 t.	Powdered Jamestown (jimson) seeds
1 t.	Boar's tusk root[98] (soaked in water)

INSTRUCTIONS: beat well together. Moisten with water from which the root was taken. Apply night and morning to draw out the cancer. Do not force detachment of the slough as this could permit the roots of the tumor to remain in the supporting tissue. If the slough does fall off before the roots have been destroyed, an inflammation will occur within eight to ten days. If this happens, repeat Step One every ten days until all the roots are destroyed. The plaster will then promote healing of the sore.

Pipsissewa Tea
(Chimaphila umbellata)

INSTRUCTIONS: apply a strong decoction of pipsissewa [99] tea to painful or ulcerated sores. Repeat (probably for several weeks) until healed. May leave a scar.

1734 Virginia Formula

6 oz. Sassafras root
6 oz. Dogwood root

INSTRUCTIONS: begin with one gallon of water, add herbs, boil until the mixture reduces to one pint in volume. Apply to gauze and drench the affected area with the decoction. Be very persistent. Drink sassafras tea in the mornings until the treatment is completed. This procedure was probably used on masses that had ulcerated. [100]

Warning: *this recipe is controversial because of adverse (and probably irrelevant) findings in relationship to sassafras and cancer.*

DR. SAMUEL THOMSON
1769–1843

Cancer Plaster

Red clover blossoms

INSTRUCTIONS: boil the red clover blossoms in water for one hour. Many sources say to harvest the blossoms in the morning before the sun has hit them. To prevent burning, a double boiler is recommended. Remove the blossoms, but not the liquid. Fill the kettle with fresh blossoms (use the same liquid). Repeat procedure. Strain and press the heads to get out as much of the juice as possible. Then, simmer over a low heat until the expressed juice has the consistency of tar. Spread on gauze and apply directly to the tumor.

To reduce smarting, add dandelion extract.

NOTE: a variation of this procedure was reported not too long ago in newspapers in Ohio. Someone put wood sorrel in a large barrel, filled it with water, and left the mixture in the sun. This turned to a tar-like consistency and was apparently successfully applied as an escharotic paste. Wood sorrel belongs to the same family of herbs as red clover.

DR. J. WELDON FELL
Middlesex Hospital 1858

The Fell Remedy[101]

Root of puccoon plant (bloodroot)
Chloride of zinc

JOHN PATTISON [102]
1866

Enucleating Paste[103]

EQUAL PARTS

Hydrastis canadensis (goldenseal)
Chloride of zinc
Flour
Water

Calendula Ointment[104]

No formula provided

JOHN GOODALE BRIANTE
1870

Cancer Cure[105]

"King of all Poisons"[106]

Pound, pulverize, and bind to the cancer. It will take out the inflammation. Then use a wash: take hard-wood ashes, leach them, boil down the liquor until it is very strong. Apply twice a day with a swab to kill the cancer.

Was-a-mo-s Syrup

ROOTS OF :	HERBS OF:
Spikenard	White vervain
Sweet fern	Pigeon cherry
Yellow dock	White pine bark
Elecampane	Sweet cicely
Bloodroot	

William Fox, M.D.
1904

Cancer Liniment

2 oz. Blue flag (*Iris versicolor*) tincture
1 oz. Red clover tincture
1 oz. Bloodroot tincture

INSTRUCTIONS: mix thoroughly. Saturate a cloth and apply to the affected area. Cover with plastic to retain moisture. Change dressings twice a day.

Dr. Eli G. Jones, M.D.
1911

These formulae were published in *Cancer: Its Causes, Symptoms and Treatment*.

Jones used a form of annotation unfamiliar to herbalists today. The symbol following zinc chloride is for a troy ounce (480 grains or 28.3495 grams.) I believe that "a.a." stands for "as above" and "iiss" for two ounces, semis, half of each. I believe this to mean that the formula calls for two ounces of the chlorides, half of each. The first formula is not therefore as aggressive as some.

Paste No. 1

FOR USE ON RESIDUAL MALIGNANCY AFTER THE ESCHAR HAS DETACHED

1 oz. Saturated solution of chromium chloride
1 oz. Saturated solution of zinc chloride
6 oz. Solid extract sanguinaria
6 oz. Pulverized sanguinaria
1 oz   Glycerine

INSTRUCTIONS: prepare as needed since the paste tends to harden. Dr. Jones remarked that this is the least painful of the pastes but that it does not go deep enough. Therefore, he recommended using it after a growth has already been removed and the sore is healing. It will stimulate the tissue to become active when healing is occurring too quickly or reactions are slow. He suggested wetting a camel's hair brush in the solution and dabbing it on the site two or three times. This is enough to stimulate the process and keep the treatment going when the process is slowing down.

Paste No. 2

FOR SMALL SKIN CANCERS UPON THE NOSE AND FOREHEAD

1 dram   Pulverized galangal root
1 dram   Zinc chloride
1/2 dram Starch
          Enough water to make a paste

A dram is 60 grains, 1/8 troy ounce. The notation system is unfamiliar to modern herbalists.

Paste No. 3

4 drams	Solid extract sanguinaria (alcoholic)
12 drams	Zinc chloride
1 dram	Starch
2 drams	Red saunders

NOTE: use soft sanguinaria, not the dry solid extract. Alternatively, water can be added to soften the paste, or more pulverized sanguinaria can be added to thicken it.

Paste No. 4

FOR BREAST CANCER

TO PASTE NO. 3, ADD EQUAL PARTS:

Saturated solution of zinc chloride
25% solution of carbolic acid

INSTRUCTIONS: add this to Paste No. 3 to soften it. Use this paste where the condition is ulcerated and where it is necessary to penetrate deeply to reach the bottom of the diseased mass. This is often the case with certain advanced breast tumors.

NOTE: Dr. Jones had his own method of application of the escharotics. He placed adhesive strips around the affected area to prevent the pastes from making contact with healthy tissue.

Then, he spread the paste onto a soft white cloth the size of the exposed area and pressed it onto the malignant area with a wad of absorbent cotton. He next covered this with adhesive strips to keep the cloth in place. He changed dressings every twenty-four hours and bathed the surface with warm water. He continued these applications until the patient reported a feeling of a heavy, dead weight. Then, he switched to a poultice.

Poultice Powder

EQUAL PARTS:

Pulverized slippery elm
Pulverized flax seed
Pulverized lobelia seed
Pulverized bayberry bark

INSTRUCTIONS: put 1-2 teaspoons of the powder into a container, add enough boiling water to make a poultice. Stir until the lumps disappear; spread onto a soft white cloth large enough to cover the growth and the inflamed area around the growth. Repeat every two hours. Bathe the skin around the growth with equal parts distilled witch hazel and warm water each time the poultice is changed. When the growth breaks loose and drops onto the poultice, examine the area to see if it looks healthy. If so, apply the yellow healing salve. If not, continue with the poultice.

Yellow Healing Salve

EQUAL PARTS:

Burgundy pitch
White pine turpentine
Beeswax
Mutton tallow
Olive oil

INSTRUCTIONS: melt, stir, and cool. Then, add 5 parts cosmoline.[107] Spread onto soft white cloth and apply three times a day. It will draw out the unhealthy pus. If it draws too hard and causes smarting or pain, add one part Vaseline to three parts salve and apply as before.

The above "yellow healing salve" I have used in all the years of my practice and I have never found anything to equal it.[108]

Compound Syrup Scrophularia

32 oz.	Scrophularia (leaves and roots)
8 oz.	Phytolacca root
8 oz.	Rumex crispus root
4 oz.	Celastrus scandens bark and root
2 oz.	Corydalis formosa root
4 oz.	Podophyllum root
3 oz.	Juniper berries
1 oz.	Prickly ash berries
2 oz.	Guiacum wood
	Oil of sassafras

INSTRUCTIONS: use fresh herbs. Mix. Coarsely bruise the herbs. Moisten with dilute alcohol and let stand for two or three days. Place in a steam displacement apparatus and pass through the vapor of three pints of alcohol; continue this displacement with the steam of water until the strength is exhausted. Set aside the three pints of tincture that passed first and evaporate the remainder to two pints. Mix these together and add 6 pints of syrup (Ovi). Add oil of sassafras, as much as necessary, to flavor.

DOSE: one tablespoon three times a day or enough to keep the bowels regular.

"It has been the earnest study of my life to find such a combination which I could leave as a help to my brother physicians in their efforts to cure the more desperate forms of this disease. I have the utmost faith in the curative power of this combination . . . great care should be taken to get fresh herbs to make the syrup."[109]

FREDERIC E. MOHS, B.Sc., M.D.
1910–

Zinc Chloride Fixative Paste[110]

40.0 gm	Stibnite
	(sifted through 80 mesh sieve)
10.0 gm	*Sanguinaria canadensis*
34.5 ml	Zinc chloride, saturated solution

DIRECTIONS: thoroughly mix stibnite and sanguinaria in the dry state. Add zinc chloride to produce a paste of the proper consistency. Zinc chloride makes up about 40-50% of the preparation by weight.

Harry S. Hoxsey
1901–1974

Though I do not subscribe to the proprietary zeal with which the Hoxsey family guarded its cancer recipes, I recognize their dedication to the treatment methods. Hoxsey spent a large part of his life fighting legal battles over the formulae. In the end, prestigious panels of medical investigators and two Federal courts upheld the therapeutic benefits of the formulae; in fact, the Hoxsey treatment was deemed clinically superior to surgery, chemotherapy, and radiation; but these findings did not spare Hoxsey from further persecution. His chain of clinics in the United States was eventually closed and a new clinic was opened in Tijuana in the late 1950's.

Hoxsey believed that the yellow powder was selective and only acted on malignant tissue but that the paste and liquid (acid) are not selective. The spread of these was managed by "erecting a vaseline or zinc oxide fence around the area to be treated."[111] In fact, Hoxsey believed that the escharotic triggers a chain reaction extending an inch or two beyond the place of application.

Trichloroacetic acid

The Hoxsey Escharotic Salve

Antimony trisulfide
Zinc chloride
Bloodroot

Black Pills

75 mg.	Potassium iodide
10 mg.	Licorice
10 mg.	Red clover
5 mg.	Burdock root
5 mg.	Stillingia root
5 mg.	Berberis root
5 mg.	Poke root
5 mg.	Cascara amarga
2.5 mg.	Prickly ash bark
10 mg.	Buckthorn bark

DOSE: two pills, four times per day.

Red Pills

75 mg.	Potassium iodide
10 mg.	Red clover
5 mg.	Stillingia root
5 mg.	Berberis root
5 mg.	Poke root
10 mg.	Buckthorn bark
1/10 mg.	Pepsin

DOSE: two pills, four times per day.

Yellow Powder

Arsenic trisulfide   (WARNING: *poisonous.*)
Sublimed sulphur
Antimony trisulfide (According to court records.)

OTHER SOURCES: include elder blossoms (*Sambucus canadensis*), bloodroot (*Sanguinaria canadensis*), and magnolia flowers (*Magnolia glauca)*, talc, and "yellow precipitate," possibly *arsenic trisulfide* (i.e. redundant) or sulfur.

THE INGREDIENTS LISTED ARE FROM COURT RECORDS AND OTHER PUBLISHED SOURCES THAT ARE NOT ENTIRELY CLEAR BECAUSE OF DUPLICATIONS AND INCONSISTENCIES.

TRIFOLIUM COMPOUND

The following formula is the one used by Hoxsey, made public following FDA analysis of Elixirex. It is my firm belief that this recipe was popular long before Hoxsey's family came into possession of it. After many years use of an essentially identical blood purifying formula, Dr. John Christopher discovered that a medicine man for whom he had the highest regard employed a similar tonic. Chief Sundance was from Idaho Falls and claimed to have received the recipe via divine inspiration. Hoxsey obtained his recipe on the deathbed of his grandfather, Christopher after trial and error using traditional recipes. My own suspicion is that the formula and concepts governing its use are Native American, that they were appropriated by the Eclectic physicians and modified by individual practitioners according to availability of the ingredients and patient needs.

REVIEW BY E. EDGAR BOND, M.D. [112]

After many years, Hoxsey's formulae were chemically analyzed and peer reviewed. The conclusion was that the approach was not "shotgun" but rather many sided, that the preparations are alteratives, blood builders, mildly stimulating so that the system is urged to eliminate pathological accumulations and rebuild, that the protocol addressed the systemic nature of the disease rather than focusing on the local manifestations of cancer.

Hoxsey Tonic

AMOUNT/5 CC	AMOUNT IN 16 OZ. BOTTLE
30 parts	Potassium iodide (150 mg)
4 parts	Buckthorn bark (20 mg)
4 parts	Licorice root (20 mg)
4 parts	Red clover blossoms (20 mg)
2 parts	Barberry root (10) mg
2 parts	Burdock root (10 mg)
2 parts	Poke root (10 mg)
	(do not exceed dosage)
2 parts	Stillingia root (10 mg)
1 part	Cascara sagrada (5 mg)
1 part	Prickly ash bark (5 mg)

INSTRUCTIONS: prepare into a liquid and add honey drip cane. The recommended maximum dosage is one teaspoonful, four times per day; some patients may want to start with smaller amounts and work up to the therapeutic levels.

COMMENTS: since this recipe has been the object of greed, lawsuits, and secrecy, some discussion is probably appropriate.

According to Jonathan L. Hartwell, most of the herbs in the formulae have anticancer action: barberry, buckthorn, burdock, cascara sagrada, red clover, licorice, poke root, and prickly ash.[113] Originally, Hoxsey apparently used bloodroot (which is also antitumoral) in the elixir. Later, bloodroot was only used in the external salve. Mildred Nelson, head of the clinic in Mexico that has continued the work of Hoxsey, has substituted chaparral for poke root. Though the reports are not entirely credible, Hoxsey claimed to vary the formula according to individual patient requirements. Instructions often stated that the elixir was to be used so long as bowel movements remained tar-like.

Dr. John R. Christopher
1909-1983

These are formulae described by the late Dr. John R. Christopher in his lectures and books[114] as well as by Sam Biser in *The Layman's Course on Killing Cancer*, material based on the work of Dr. Christopher.

Anticancer Remedy[115]

BASIC TRIFOLIUM COMPOUND, SIMILAR TO HOXSEY'S TONIC, ALSO CALLED "BLACK DOGWOOD TEA"

EQUAL PARTS:

Red clover blossoms	Burdock root
Poke root	Buckthorn bark
Licorice root	Stillingia root
Cascara sagrada	Oregon grape root
Sarsaparilla root	Peach bark
Prickly ash bark	Chaparral leaves

PREPARATION: 1 tsp. to one cup; infuse with boiling water. Take 1/3 cup 3 times per day. Increase by 1/3 cup every three weeks until reaching one cup three times a day.

VARIATIONS AND NOTES: in some places, Christopher does not mention cascara sagrada or sarsaparilla in this formula. In others, he adds alfalfa and sometimes also peach bark and Oregon grape root. He did not use potassium iodide, but he subscribed to the view that it is much needed in cancer prevention. Dr. Max Gerson did use potassium iodide in his cancer treatment. Herbalists often use large amounts of Irish moss instead of potassium iodide. Native Americans used ashes that might have had a very similar effect. Christopher's formula was made into a tea. He recommended drinking three cups of tea per day, six days a week until feeling more "pep and energy." After a course of treatment, usually six weeks, patients were often advised to switch to burdock, chaparral, or Brigham tea. Later, they were to take red clover again.

Red Sun Balm—Cayenne Salve[116]

AN ESCHAROTIC THAT CAN ALSO BE USED FOR ARTHRITIS, MUSCLE SORENESS, STIFF NECK, SPRAINS AND BRUISES

Cayenne pepper (African bird pepper)
Olive oil
Oil of wintergreen
Pure distilled mint crystals
Untreated beeswax

COMMENTS: in some places, these same ingredients are listed along with the comment "other herbal oils." The salve is used in a manner similar to the escharotic salves. It stimulates circulation while the *Black Ointment* draws out the toxins. Christopher sometimes recommended applying the pastes on top of each other as well as alternating them.

Attention: this is the escharotic salve whereas the Black Ointment is the drawing salve. Black Ointment is not an escharotic.

German Kermesberro—
Black ointment [117]

THIS PREPARATION CAN BE USED, INDE-
PENDENTLY OF THE CAYENNE SALVE, ON
ULCERS, BOILS, WARTS, BURNS, HEMOR-
RHOIDS, SKIN CANCERS, AND TUMORS.

1.5 pounds	Mutton tallow

I POUND OF FRESH OR HALF POUND OF DRY HERBS
OF EACH OF THE FOLLOWING:

> Chaparral
> Red clover blossoms
> Comfrey root
> Plantain
> Chickweed
> Poke root
> Mullein

ADD:

1 oz.	Beeswax
3-4 oz.	Olive oil
1/4 pint	Pine tar

INSTRUCTIONS: melt the tallow in a stainless steel pot at 170°F in an oven. Discard cracklings, add herbs, and put in oven for 3-4 hours. Remove, strain, and warm once more. Add beeswax, olive oil, and pine tar. Use a beater to homogenize and pour into wide mouthed jar.

SUBSTITUTIONS: like most herbalists, Christopher recognized that many herbs have similar properties so that where certain herbs are not available, substitutions can be made. He also advised that where some ingredients are lacking, it is better to use the ones on hand, i.e. a partial formula, rather than to wait and do nothing. In one source, he gave a slightly different version of this formula that included kino, wheat germ oil, glycerine (2 oz.), goldenseal, and marshmallow root. In another, licorice was listed as an ingredient.

Poke Root Poultice (Phytolacca)

FOR BREAST CANCER

> Fresh green poke root
> Fluid extract poke root
> Apple cider vinegar
> Bayberry root powder

DIRECTIONS: grind fresh poke, sufficient for one application. Roll onto a piece of muslin or gauze; cut hole large enough for the nipple. Apply to the breast; moisten with fluid extract phytolacca and cover with plastic to retain moisture. Leave on for three days; then apply fresh poultice. In two weeks the breast will break out in pustular sores; in four weeks, all hardness will be gone. When this occurs, wash thoroughly with apple cider vinegar; cover with bayberry powder and allow the entire breast surface to dry. In 7-10 days, the entire surface will be healed. [118]

INSTRUCTIONS: use together with black dogwood tea (the "anticancer remedy") and elderberry tincture. Will remove cysts and tumors.

Fomentation for Breast Cancer

3 parts	Mullein
1 part	Lobelia

INSTRUCTIONS: use internally and externally.

Herbal Bolus

FOR TUMORS OF THE COLON AS WELL AS
THE MALE AND FEMALE REPRODUCTIVE
SYSTEMS. CAN ALSO BE USED FOR CERVICAL
DYSPLASIA, HYPERPLASIA, PRECANCEROUS
CONDITIONS, AND CANDIDA ALBICANS

USE EQUAL PARTS OF THE FOLLOWING HERBS

Squaw vine   Goldenseal root
Chickweed   Mullein leaves
Slippery elm bark   Marshmallow root
Comfrey root   Yellow dock root
Cocoa butter

INSTRUCTIONS: since herbs powder differently, grind each herb separately. Blend the powders. Melt the cocoa butter in a crock pot or double boiler. As soon as the cocoa butter has lique-fied, stir the herbs into the cocoa butter and mix thoroughly. Allow the herbs to cook in the cocoa butter for about twenty minutes.[119] Stir continuously and be careful that the herbs do not burn. After twenty minutes, unplug the crock pot and allow the mixture to cool. As the consistency becomes thicker, watch care-fully. When it is firm enough to shape, yet still malleable, shape into suppositories the thick-ness of a pencil or finger. Make them an inch to an inch-and-a-half long, wrap individually in wax paper, and store in the refrigerator until needed.

USE: insert vaginally and/or rectally, as indi-cated, before bedtime daily or every other day six days each week until symptoms disappear. Use a douche or enema before inserting a fresh bolus.

Vaginal Douche

CAN ALSO BE USED FOR PROLAPSES

6 parts	Oak bark
3 parts	Mullein
4 parts	Yellow dock
3 parts	Walnut bark or leaves
6 parts	Comfrey root
1 part	Lobelia
3 parts	Squaw vine

INSTRUCTIONS: use pure water, preferably dis-tilled water. Simmer until the water has reduced, approximately half an hour or until the brew is quite strong, cover, and allow to cool. When body temperature, inject 1/4 to 1/2 cup of the tea with a syringe into the vagina. Retain the tea twenty minutes or as long as comfortable. If you have a slant board or can rig up a sloping surface, it will help to retain the fluid and deliver it where needed. Gentle massaging of the abdominal area while reclining will also improve results.

NOTE: This preparation can also be consumed as a tea. Use one part concoction to three parts distilled water.

Herbal Enema

CAN BE USED BY THOSE WITH PROSTATE OR COLON CANCER

Use the above douche formula, but substitute marshmallow root for squaw vine.

INSTRUCTIONS: prepare as above. It should be used as an enema.

NOTE: This preparation can also be consumed as a tea. Use one part concoction to three parts distilled water.

DOSE: three cups per day.

Tea #1: Squaw Vine Tea[120]

TO HARMONIZE HORMONES OF BOTH THE MALE AND FEMALE REPRODUCTIVE SYSTEMS

EQUAL PARTS

Squaw vine	Sarsaparilla
Licorice root	Siberian ginseng
Black cohosh	False unicorn root
Blessed thistle	

COMMENTS: Dr. Christopher recommended this tea for hormonal fluctuations at the change of life or when there is stress on or a disturbance to the reproductive system: puberty, pregnancy, childbirth, and menopause. Squaw vine contains natural hormonal precursors that regulate hormonal balance so that abnormal growths and difficult and irregular periods are corrected.

DOSAGE: 1-3 tablets or capsules or one cup of tea morning and evening.

Female Reproductive System[121]

CIRCULATORY FORMULA

3 parts	Goldenseal
1 part	Blessed thistle
1 part	Cayenne
1 part	Cramp bark
1 part	False unicorn root
1 part	Jamaican ginger
1 part	Red raspberry leaves
1 part	Squaw vine
1 part	Uva ursi leaves

INSTRUCTIONS FOR TINCTURE: place one ounce of herb mixture in a jar, add four ounces of grain alcohol and seal. Shake daily for fourteen days. Strain.

DOSAGE: 10-20 drops in water three times a day.

TEA: use the same ingredients to make a tea. Drink one cup of tea morning and evening for six days each week for 90-120 days.

CAPSULES: take two "O" size capsules each morning and evening for six days each week for 90-120 days.

NOTE: Dr. Christopher always recommended suspending use of herbs one day each week.

COMMENTS: this formula compliments the squaw vine tea and should be used in conjunction with it.

This formula stimulates circulation, particularly in the reproductive system. It relieves painful menstruation due to congestion. In his lectures, Dr. Christopher stated that the herbs in this formula help to strengthen and rebuild the female reproductive organs: the uterus, ovaries, and fallopian tubes. He also said it relieves cramps, hot flashes, leukorrhea, yeast infections, anemia, as well as painful and swollen breasts.

Male Reproductive System[122]

CIRCULATORY FORMULA. TO CLEAN OUT SEDIMENTATION, MUCUS, AND INFECTION IN THE PROSTATE

Cayenne
Jamaican ginger
Goldenseal
Gravel root or queen of the meadow root
Juniper berries
Marshmallow root
Parsley root
Uva ursi leaves
Siberian ginseng

DOSAGE: 2-3 capsules, "O" size, mornings and evenings with parsley root tea, a mucusless diet, distilled water, and fresh juices.

INSTRUCTIONS: use the lower bowel formula first. Then, "because cancer has a difficult time growing in the presence of organic potassium," use black walnuts or elderberries or other foods high in potassium. Also use the partridge berry (squaw vine) to increase hormonal production to restore the gland.

Cancerous Growths[123]

EQUAL PARTS
Red clover
Violet
Burdock root
Yellow dock
Dandelion root
Rock rose
Goldenseal root

INSTRUCTIONS: infuse in boiling water; let set until cool enough to drink. One wineglassful three times a day.

RENÉE CAISSE
1888-1978

Essiac Formula

PARTS BY WEIGHT

24 oz.	Burdock, cut and dried
16 oz.	Indian rhubarb root, powdered
4 oz.	Slippery elm inner bark, powdered
1 oz.	Sheep's sorrel, powdered

Many bulk herb packages (to be prepared as teas) and tinctures containing these ingredients are available in health foods stores. It should be noted that Caisse administered her remedy both as a tea and intravenously. Later in her life, Caisee added four more herbs:

2 oz.	Kelp
1 oz.	Red clover
1 oz.	Blessed thistle
.4 oz.	Watercress

SUPPLIES: 4 gallon stainless steel pot with lid, 3 gallon stainless steel pot with lid, stainless steel double strainer, funnel and spatula, 12 or more 16 oz. amber bottles.

INSTRUCTIONS: Mix dry ingredients thoroughly. Put in plastic bag and shake vigorously. Store in cool, dark place. Use the four gallon pot. Bring two gallons of sodium free distilled water to boil; stir in one cup of ingredients. Put the lid on the pot and boil for ten minutes. Turn off heat. Scrape down sides of pot with spatula and stir. Replace the lid.

Allow the pot to remain closed for twelve hours. Turn on the heat to the highest setting and allow the brew to come almost to the boiling point. Do not boil. Turn off the heat. Strain into the three gallon pot. Clean the four gallon pot and strainer. Pour the liquid through the strainer into the four gallon pot. Use the funnel to pour the hot tea into sterilized bottles. Tighten the caps on the bottles. Check again for tightness after the jars have cooled. Refrigerate.

DOSE: Shake before using. Take two ounces at bedtime, at least two hours after eating.

MISCELLANEOUS PREPARATIONS

Sichert's Lymphatic Ointment

THIS IS USED FOR LYMPHOEDEMA, ESPECIALLY FOLLOWING MASTECTOMIES.

EXTRACTS OF:

Hemlock	Foxglove
Henbane	Autumn crocus
May apple	

INSTRUCTIONS: massage firmly twice daily. More effective if used in conjunction with Vodder's manual lymphatic drainage therapy and compression bandages.

Super Draw Poultice

handful	Red clover blossoms
	Fresh raw organic garlic
	(amount depends on sensitivity of
	the treatment area)
a few T.	Charcoal
a few T	Bentonite clay
a few T	Poke root
a few T.	Slippery elm powder
	Apple cider vinegar
	(raw organic)
	Water

Proportions are "intuitive." Put ingredients into blender and add liquids to make the right consistency. The poultice should be moist, not runny. It will become gelatinous fairly quickly because of the slippery elm. It should be applied immediately. It can be applied directly to the skin or to a soft gauze. It should be held in place by a waterproof dressing. The poultice should be changed if it dries out, if it becomes odorous, or if visual inspection indicates that it has absorbed morbid matter or changed color.

Chaparral

DOSE: go on a strong regime for a short time: six tablets or capsules a day for three weeks. If you can stand the taste and smell, you can drink chaparral as a tea.

CA25 Blood Cleanser

BLOOD PURIFYING FORMULA FOR NEUTRALIZING AND REMOVING TOXINS

INCLUDES TWENTY-FIVE HERBS:

Echinacea, red clover, plantain, chaparral, artemisia, blue flag, pau d'arco, oak bark, dandelion, burdock, sheep's sorrel, cascara sagrada, buckthorn, Oregon grape root, sassafras, sarsaparilla, gentian.

Dose: 2-3 capsules, two or three times a day.

Source: Chad Van Seters from his father Joseph Van Seters.

Jason Winters Tea

Red clover
Chaparral
Cayenne

The Black and Yellow Salves and Related Escharotics

The formulae for the two salves mentioned by Jane Heimlich as having been used by Dr. H. Ray Evers have not been confirmed. My sense is that most "black salve" and "compound X" formulae are more or less traditional though each producer tends to have his or her own variations. They are both, of course, pastes rather than salves. However, most "black salves" are used in conjunction with yellow salves whereas most "compound X" preparations are stand alone treatments that are also often used internally whereas the "black salves" are seldom recommended for internal use.

Compound X

Virxcan

Bloodroot	Red clover
Burdock root	Sheep's sorrel
Turmeric	Calcium phosphate
Polymer of castor bean	
Zinc chloride	
"An herb from Taiwan"	

Use: externally as an escharotic salve or diluted as a douche: 1/2 teaspoon to one quart water. It is also available in tablets for internal use. This is not the complete formula, but these ingredients have been confirmed by the manufacturer. Certain batches are made with greater celandine, *Chelidonium major*, instead of bloodroot.

Source: Mark Currie

Black Salve

PROPORTIONS BY WEIGHT:
25% Galangal root
25% Bloodroot
50% Zinc chloride

Instructions: put the zinc chloride (99.4% pure) in an uncovered glass bowl. Depending on heat and humidity, it may take as long as four days to liquefy. Adding distilled water will promote faster liquefaction. Grind the herbs; being careful to keep the temperature below 100F. Add the herbs to the zinc chloride and stir thoroughly. At first, the mixture will be a bit thin. Add flour to thicken to the consistency of toothpaste. The pH should be in the 3.7-3.8 range. If not, add more powdered herbs in equal proportions.

Note: do not use metal with zinc chloride. Be sure to add the herbs to the zinc chloride rather than vice versa and stir with a wooden utensil.

Source: Dan Raber

Raber supports use of this external treatment with internal remedies. He puts powdered bloodroot and galangal in capsules and uses 20-30 drops of bloodroot tincture per day. He obeys the Christopher rule of suspending treatment one day per week. He states that the paste is absorbed very rapidly as after application to a treatment site, it can be tasted in the mouth within a few seconds. He also noted that some practitioners are adding pine tar and echinacea to their pastes.

Escharotic Black Salve

PERCENT BY WEIGHT

Distilled water 25.0%
Zinc chloride 34.0
Chaparral 4:1 7.5
Bloodroot concentrate 14.0
Cayenne 6.0
Glycerine U.S.P. 3.0
Red clover 4:1 2.0
Turmeric 4:1 5.0
Dimethylsulfoxide (DMSO) 2.0
Burdock root 4:1 1.0
Citric acid 0.5

Thicken with FMC SeaKem GP-317 (Irish Moss) if necessary. DMSO must be pharmaceutical grade. Cayenne should have a Scoville rating of 40,000 or greater.

PROCEDURE: dissolve the zinc chloride in the warm distilled water. Blend all the herbal powders and bloodroot in a separate container. Slowly add the zinc chloride solution to the herbal blend while stirring. Mix well. Add the glycerine and citric acid and mix thoroughly. Gently heat this mixture in an oven at 120°F for approximately eight hours. Remove from heat, stir well, and allow to cool. The process requires curing. Either let the mixture sit for one week or force cure in oven.

SOURCE: Dan Ostrander

C-Herb

AN ESCHAROTIC PRODUCT

White oak bark
Burdock
Black walnut
Fiber
Mineral salts
"Other well known herbs"
Water

SOURCE: John H. Berge

The Yellow Salve

Mutton tallow
Linseed oil
Beeswax
Oil of wintergreen
Oil of spike

USE: to be used in accordance with the directions provided by the producer. This salve has also been reported to be useful in the treatment of herpes.

SOURCE: Ken Michaelis

Enucleating Salve à la Pattison

A basic enucleating salve suitable for ulcerated conditions. It is almost painless, but not aggressive. Zinc chloride can be added to increase the strength.

PARTS BY WEIGHT:

5 oz.	Goldenseal
4 oz.	Turmeric
3 oz.	White willow bark
	Calendula oil
	Calendula CO_2

INSTRUCTIONS: use enough calendula oil (made in apricot kernel oil) to make a thick preparation, somewhat the same consistency as toothpaste. Cure overnight in a yoghurt maker or other appliance that will maintain an even temperature of 98-105°F.

Ingrid's Golden Myrrical

Useful to keep the treatment site from closing prematurely.

PARTS BY WEIGHT:

5 oz.	Goldenseal
4 oz.	Myrrh
3 oz.	Irish moss
	Castor oil
	Calendula CO_2

INSTRUCTIONS: use enough castor oil to blend all the powders. The mixture should be quite thick. Cure overnight in a yoghurt maker.

Coptis Fomentation

To remove heat from the breast or liver

Coptis

INSTRUCTIONS: make a strong decoction (like a tea) of coptis. Do not boil, but let the herbs steep in very hot water for at least 20 minutes. Refrigerate what is not immediately needed. Saturate a clean cloth or sterile gauze with the fomentation and apply to the affected area. Replace the dressing if it becomes dry. Continue so long as the area has excess heat.

Cleavers Tea

5 oz.	Cleavers
3.5 oz.	Ginger, cut and sifted
3 oz.	Sarsaparilla pieces
3 oz.	Chinese licorice pieces
2 oz.	Star anise pieces
2 oz.	Cardamom pods, broken
1 oz.	Galangal, cut and sifted
1 oz.	Orange peels
1 oz.	Black peppercorns, broken
1/4 oz.	Cloves, broken

INSTRUCTIONS: put larger pieces into a coffee mill or blender to break slightly. Blend ingredients. Use in a tea infuser and steep 10-20 minutes before drinking.

Poultice à la Jones

For use on open areas with discharge or inflamed sites.

EQUAL PARTS OF THE POWDERED HERBS:

Coptis
Slippery elm bark
Flax seed
Lobelia leaf
Bayberry root bark

INSTRUCTIONS: stir the herbs together. Separate out enough for one application, usually only a spoonful. Add warm, purified water. The mixture will swell up quickly and become somewhat mucilaginous. Apply to the affected area and cover with a clean cloth, clean leaves (such as cabbage or basil), or waterproof material. Change at least every 24 hours or whenever the dressing becomes dry or odorous.

Carminative Capsules

For digestion and elimination

4 oz.	Psyllium husks
2 oz.	Orange peel
2 oz.	Cascara sagrada
2 oz.	Oregon grape root
2 oz.	Gentian
1.5 oz.	Star anise
3 T.	Ginger
1 T.	Cinnamon
2 t.	Cardamom
1 t.	Cayenne

DIRECTIONS: fill "00" vegetarian gelatin capsules and take one to six capsules per day as needed.

Common & Botanical Names

COMMON NAME INDEX

Alfalfa	*Medicago sativa*	Comfrey	*Symphytum officinale*
American ginseng	*Panax quinquefolium*	Coptis	*Coptis chinensis*
American mandrake	*Podophyllum peltatum*	Cramp bark	*Viburnum opulus*
Barberry	*Berberis vulgaris*	Dandelion	*Taraxacum officinale*
Basil	*Osymum basilicum*	Duckweed	*Lemna minor*
Bayberry	*Myrica cerifera*	Elder	*Sambucus nigra*
Bearberry	*Arctostaphylos uva-ursi*	Elecampane	*Inula helenium*
Black cohosh	*Cimicifuga racemosa*	False unicorn	*Helonias dioica*
Blessed thistle	*Cnicus benedictus*	Fennel	*Foeniculum vulgare*
Bloodroot	*Sanguinaria canadensis*	Field mustard	*Sinapis arvenis*
Blue flag	*Iris versicolor*	Figwort	*Scrophularia nodosa*
Buckthorn	*Rhamnus frangula*	Flax seed	*Linum usitatissimum*
Burdock	*Arctium lappa*	Frankincense	*Boswellia thurifera*
Calendula	*Calendula officinalis*	Galangal	*Alpina officinarum*
Cascara sagrada	*Rhamnus purshiana*	Ginger (Jamaican)	*Zingiber officialis*
Cayenne pepper	*Capsicum annuum*	Ginseng	*Panax ginseng*
Chaparral	*Larrea divaricata*	Goldenseal	*Hydrastis canadensis*
Chickweed	*Stellaria media*	Gotu kola	*Hydrocotyle asiatica*
Cinnamon, Ceylon	*Cinamomum zeylanicum / verum*	Gravel root	*Eupatorium purpureum*
		Guggulu	*Commiphora mukul*
Climbing bittersweet	*Celastrus scandens*	Guaiacum wood	*Guaiacum officinale*

Holy thistle	*Cnicus benedictus*	Sheep's sorrel	*Rumex acetosa*
Indian rhubarb	*Rheum palmatum*	Siberian ginseng	*Eleutherococcus sentiosus*
Irish moss	*Chondrus crispus*	Slippery elm	*Ulmus fulva*
Jimson weed	*Datura stramonium*	Spikenard	*Aralia racemosa*
Juniper	*Juniperus communis*	Squaw vine	*Mitchella repens*
Kino	*Pterocarpus marsupium*	Staff vine	*Celastrus scandens*
Licorice	*Glycyrrhiza glabra*	Stillingia	*Stillingia sylvatica*
Lobelia	*Lobelia inflata*	Sweet cicely	*Myrrhis odorata*
Magnolia	*Magnolia acuminata*	Sweet fern	*Comptonia Peregrina*
Mandrake	*Atropa mandragora*	Thuja	*Thuja occidentalis*
May apple	*Podophyllum peltatum*	Tormentil	*Potentilla tormentilla*
Marshmallow	*Althaea officinalis*	Trichosanthes	*Trichosanthes kirilowii*
Milk thistle	*Carduus marianus*	Turkey corn	*Corydalis formosa*
Mullein	*Verbascum thapsus*	Turmeric	*Curcuma longa*
Myrrh	*Commiphora myrrha*	Uva ursi	*Arctostaphylos uva-ursi*
Oak bark	*Quercus alba*	Violet	*Viola spp.*
Oregon grape root	*Mahonia repens*	Wahoo	*Euonymus atropurpureus*
Pau d'arco	*Tabebuia impetiginosa*	Walnut bark	*Juglans nigra*
Peach bark	*Amygdalis persica*	White pine	*Pinus strobus*
Pepper, black	*Piper nigrum*	White oak	*Quercus alba*
Pepper, long	*Piper longum*	White vervain	*Verbena Urticifolia*
Pepper, white	*Piper album*	Wild bedstraw	*Galium aparine*
Pipsissewa	*Chimaphila umbellata*	Wintergreen	*Gaultheria procumbens*
Plantain	*Plantago major*	Wormwood	*Artemisia absinthium*
Poke root	*Phytolacca decandra*	Yarrow	*Achillea millefolium*
Prickly ash	*Xanthoxylum americanum*	Yellow dock	*Rumex crispus*
Pseudoginseng	*Panax notoginseng*		
Red clover	*Trifolium pratense*		
Red herb root	*Phytolacca americana*		
Red raspberry	*Rubus strigosus*		
Red sandalwood	*Pterocarpus santilinus*		
Red saunders	*Pterocarpus santilinus*		
Rock rose	*Helianthemum canadense*		
Rue	*Ruta graveolens*		
Sage, garden	*Salvia officinalis*		
Sarsaparilla	*Smilax officinalis*		

Though some of these names are traditional, most of them are the ones used by Sam Biser in *The Layman's Course on Killing Cancer*—and sometimes by Dr. John Christopher.

American mandrake	May apple	King of all Poisons	(perhaps arsenic)
Arrow wood	Wahoo	Linseed	Flax seed
Bardana	Burdock	Maiden barber	Barberry
Bearberry	Uva ursi	Mandrake	May apple
Black dogwood	Buckthorn	Marigold	*Calendula officinalis*
Bladderpod	Lobelia	Moose elm	Slippery elm
Blessed thistle	Holy thistle	Nipbone	Comfrey
Boar's tusk	(perhaps burdock)	Partridge berry	Squaw vine
Cleaver grass	Red clover	Pigeon berry	*Phytolacca decandra*
Garden patience	Yellow dock	Red saunders	Red sandalwood
German Kermesberro	Poke root	Snakeweed	Plantain
		Spindle tree	Wahoo
Greasewood	Chaparral	Starwort	False unicorn root
Jacob's staff	Mullein	White mallow	Marshmallow
Jamestown weed	Jimson weed, thorn-apple	White oak	Common European oak
		Yellow parilla	Sarsaparilla

APPENDIX D

Resources

Due to the fact that the quality, price, and supply of the products described in this book change so often, a resource list is offered on the Internet at the author's Web site:

http://www.cancersalves.com/resources.html

The site is constantly updated. It is the place where new information on the salves and adjunctive formulas for cancer are posted. Frequent visits to this site are recommended for both health care practitioners and patients. In addition to herbal products, there is valuable general health information on subjects such as the role of emotions on health, the body-mind connection, and healing the whole person.

The site is also the place where letters to the author can be sent, where questions can be answered, and where information on new research, case histories, and supervised treatment can be found.

Sacred Medicine Sanctuary
P.O. Box 235
Suquamish, Washington 98392

APPENDIX E

Suggested Reading

THERE ARE MANY APPROACHES to cancer treatment besides surgery, chemotherapy, and irradiation. For a quick but responsible overview of the various alternatives, Ralph Moss, former assistant director of public affairs at Memorial Sloan-Kettering Cancer Center, provides synopses of approximately one hundred nontoxic treatments. Pelton and Walters both extend the thumbnail sketches by covering approximately thirty of the more widely available alternatives in somewhat more detail. *Third Opinion* is a guide to treatment facilities, their treatments, and costs. It also reports on the conditions that respond best to the therapies offered. Heimlich's book is not exclusively devoted to cancer, but it is easy reading, reliable, and informative, whereas the more controversial Clark provides step-by-step instructions for self-treatment and for cleaning up one's personal environment.

An Alternative Medicine Definitive Guide to Cancer is an absolute gold mine of invaluable information on the actual protocols used by holistic physicians in treating cancer.

ALTERNATIVE TREATMENTS

Clark, Hulda Regehr, *The Cure for All Cancers*, ProMotion Publishing, San Diego, 1993.

Diamond, John W. with Cowden, Lee W. and Goldberg, Burton, *An Alternative Medicine Definitive Guide to Cancer*, Future Medicine Publishing, Inc., Tiburon, 1997.

Fink, John, *Third Opinion*, 3rd Ed., Avery Publishing Group, Inc., Garden City Park, 1997.

Heimlich, Jane, *What Your Doctor Won't Tell You*, Harper Perennial, New York, 1990.

Moss, Ralph W., *Cancer Therapy: The Independent Consumer's Guide to Non-Toxic Treatment and Prevention*, Equinox Press, New York, 1992.

Pelton, Ross, R.Ph., Ph.D. and Overholser, Lee, Ph.D., *Alternatives in Cancer Therapy: The Complete Guide to Non-Traditional Treatments*, Simon & Schuster, New York, 1994.

Walters, Richard, *Options: The Alternative Cancer Therapy Book*, Avery Publishing Group, Inc., Garden City Park, 1993.

Books on Suppression of Alternative Treatments

The decision about how to treat cancer is all too often made by a physician with minimal patient involvement. Patients usually learn of alternatives after conventional methods have failed. The following books tend to be highly critical of the medical establishment and obliquely to empower the patient to opt for more holistic approaches. Access to the information in these books may bring more clarity to the truly difficult and often unsupported decision to buck the system. Certainly, it will help all concerned to develop more intelligent responses to the cancer dilemma.

Batt, Sharon, *Patient No More: The Politics of Breast Cancer*, Gynergy Books, Charlottetown, Canada, 1994.

Bird, Christopher, *The Persecution and Trial of Gaston Naessens: The True Story of the Efforts to Suppress an Alternative Treatment for Cancer, AIDS, and Other Immunologically Based Diseases*, H J Kramer Inc, Tiburon, California, 1991.

Bogdanich, Walt, *The Great White Lie: Dishonesty, Waste, and Incompetence in the Medical Community*, A Touchstone Book, New York, 1991.

Carter, James P., *Racketeering in Medicine: The Suppression of Alternatives*, Hampton Roads Publishing Company, Inc., Norfolk, 1993.

Clorfene-Casten, Liane, *Breast Cancer: Poisons, Profits, and Prevention*, Common Courage Press, Monroe, 1996.

Houston, Robert G., *Repression and Reform in the Evaluation of Alternative Cancer Therapies*, Project Cure, Washington, D.C., 1987, 1989.

Lisa, P. Joseph, *The Assault on Medical Freedom*, Hampton Roads Publishing Company, Norfolk, 1994.

Lynes, Barry, *The Healing of Cancer: The Cures—the Cover-ups and the Solution Now!*, Marcus Books, Queensville, Ontario, 1989.

Moss, Ralph W., *The Cancer Industry: The Classic Exposé on the Cancer Establishment*, Paragon House, New York, 1991.

———. *Questioning Chemotherapy*, Equinox Press, Brooklyn, 1995.

Mullins, Eustace, *Murder by Injection: The Story of the Medical Conspiracy Against America*, The National Council for Medical Research, Staunton, Virginia, 1988.

Robbins, John, *Reclaiming our Health: Exploding the Medical Myth and Embracing the Source of True Healing*, H J Kramer, Tiburon, 1996.

Stabiner, Karen, *To Dance with the Devil: The New War on Breast Cancer, Politics, Power, and People*, Delacorte Press, New York, 1997.

Wolinsky, Howard and Brune, Tom, *The Serpent on the Staff: The Unhealthy Politics of the American Medical Association*, G. P. Putnam's Son, New York, 1994.

BOOKS AND AUDIO CASSETTES ON DIET AND COOKING

There is no consensus among experts as to what might constitute an adequate diet for a person at risk of cancer nor for someone actively dealing with cancer or the side effects of conventional treatments of cancer. While no one regime may be right for everyone, the following books provide some guidance that may help many patients to improve their understanding of the need for proper eating habits.

Jochems, Ruth, *Dr. Moerman's Anti-Cancer Diet*, Avery Publishing Group, Inc., Garden City, Park, 1990.

Johari, Harish, *The Healing Cuisine: India's Art of Ayurvedic Cooking*, Healing Arts Press, Rochester, 1994.

Keane, Maureen and Chace, Daniella, *What to Eat if You Have Cancer: A Guide to Adding Nutritional Therapy to Your Treatment Plan*, Contemporary Books, Chicago, 1996.

Keim, Rachel and Smith, Ginny, *What to Eat Now: The Cancer Lifeline Cookbook*, Sasquatch Books, Seattle, 1996.

Lad, Usha and Lad, Vasant, Dr., *Ayurvedic Cooking for Self-Healing*, The Ayurvedic Press, Albuquerque, 1997.

Passwater, Richard A., Ph.D., *Cancer Prevention and Nutritional Therapies*, Keats Publishing, Inc., New Caanan, 1993.

Schechter, Steven R., N.D., *Fighting Radiation with Foods, Herbs, & Vitamins*, East West Health Books, Brookline, 1988.

Simone, Charles B., *Cancer and Nutrition: A Ten-Point Plan to Reduce Your Risk of Getting Cancer*, Avery Publishing Group, Inc., Garden City Park, 1992.

Tiwari, Maya, *Ayurveda: A Life of Balance*, Healing Arts Press, Rochester, 1995.

ALSO RECOMMENDED

Kitchen Doctor by Ingrid Naiman, four 90-minute audio cassettes.

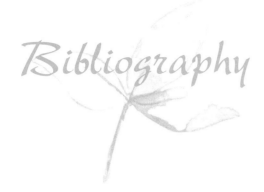

Bibliography

MEDICAL HERB BOOKS
HISTORIC

Alstat, Edward K., compiler, *Eclectic Dispensary of Botanical Therapeutics*, Eclectic Medical Publications, Portland, 1989.

Brandt, Johanna, *The Grape Cure*, Benedict Lust Publications, New York, 1928 & 1971.

Culpeper, Nicholas, *Culpeper's Complete Herbal and English Physician*, Meyerbooks, Glenwood, 1990.

David, Wm. K., *Secrets of Wise Men, Chemists, and Great Physicians*, W. K. David Publisher, Chicago, 1889.

Fox, William, M.D., *The Working Man's Model Family Botanic Guide; or Every Man His Own Doctor; Being an Exposition of the Botanic System*, Sheffield, 1904.

Grieve, M., *A Modern Herbal, Vol. I & II*, Dover Publications, Inc., New York, 1971 (originally published 1931).

Matteson, Antonette, *The Occult Family Physician and Botanic Guide to Health*, Buffalo, New York, 1894. Reprinted by Meyerbooks, Glenwood, Illinois, n.d.

Millspaugh, Charles F., *American Medicinal Plants*, Dover Publications, Inc., New York, 1974 (originally published 1892).

Meyer, Joseph E., *The Old Herb Doctor*, Hammond Book Company, 1941. Reprinted by Meyerbooks, 1993.

Potterton, David, ed., *Culpeper's Colour Herbal*, W. Foulsham & Company Limited, London, 1983.

Royle, J. Forbes, *Materia Medica and Therapeutics including Preparations of the Pharmacopœias of London, Edinburgh, Dublin, and [of the United States]*, Lea and Blanchard, Philadelphia, 1847.

Tobyn, Graeme, *Culpeper's Medicine: A Practice of Western Holistic Medicine*, Element Books Limited, Shaftesbury, 1997.

NATIVE AMERICAN FOLKLORIC USES OF HERBS

Doane, Nancy Locke, compiler, *Indian Doctor Book*, Aerial Photography Services, Inc., Charlotte, n.d.

Herrick, James W., *Iroquois Medical Botany*, Syracuse University Press, Syracuse, 1995.

Hutchens, Alma R., *Indian Herbology of North America*, Shambhala, Boston, 1991.

Murphy, Edith van Allen, *Indian Uses of Native Plants*, Mendocino County Historical Society, Ukiah, 1959 and 1987.

Stevenson, Matilda Coxe, *The Zuñi Indians and Their Uses of Plants*, First published 1908-1909. Reprinted by Dover Publications, Inc., New York, 1933.

Vogel, Virgil J., *American Indian Medicine*, University of Oklahoma Press, Norman, 1970.

Walking Night Bear, *Song of the Seven Herbs*, Book Publishing Company, Summertown, 1983.

MEDICAL HERB BOOKS MODERN

Castleman, Michael, *The Healing Herbs: The Ultimate Guide to the Curative Power of Nature's Medicines*, Rodale Press, Erasmus, 1991.

Chevallier, Andrew, *The Encyclopedia of Medicinal Plants*, DK Publishing, Inc., New York, 1996.

Christopher, Dr. John R., *School of Natural Healing*, Christopher Publications, Inc., Springville, 1983.

_____. *Dr. Christopher's Three-Day Cleansing Program, Mucusless Diet and Herbal Combinations*, Self Published, Revised Edition 1978.

Elkins, Rita, *Goldenseal*, Woodland Publishing, Pleasant Grove, 1996.

Erasmus, Udo, *Fats and Oils*, Alive Books, Vancouver, 1986.

Hall, Dorothy, *Dorothy Hall's Herbal Medicine*, Lothian Publishing Company Pty Ltd, Sydney, 1988.

Heinerman, John, *The Complete Book of Spices: Their Medical, Nutritional and Cooking Uses*, Keats Publishing, New Canaan, 1983.

Hoffman, David, editor, *The Information Sourcebook of Herbal Medicine*, The Crossing Press, Freedom, 1994.

Holmes, Peter, *The Energetics of Western Herbs, Vol. I & II*, Revised Second Edition, Artemis, Boulder, 1989, 1993.

Keville, Kathi, *Herbs for Health and Healing: A Drug-Free Guide to Prevention and Cure*, Rodale Press, Inc., Emmaus, 1996.

Kenner, Dan and Requena, Yves, *Botanical Medicine: A European Professional Perspective*, Paradigm Publications, Brookline, 1996.

Lewis, Walter H. and Elvin-Lewis, Memory P. F., *Medical Botany: Plants Affecting Man's Health*, John Wiley & Sons, New York, 1977.

Majeed, Muhammed, Ph. D., and Badmaev, Vladimir, M.D., Ph.D. and Murray, Frank, *Turmeric and the Healing Curcuminoids*, Keats Publishing, Inc., New Canaan, 1996.

Moore, Michael, *Medicinal Plants of the Desert and Canyon West*, Museum of New Mexico Press, Santa Fe, 1989.

———. *Medicinal Plants of the Mountain West*, Museum of New Mexico Press, Santa Fe, 1979.

Moss, Ralph W., *Herbs Against Cancer: History and Controversy*, Equinox Press, Brooklyn, 1998.

Mowrey, Daniel B., Ph.D., *Herbal Tonic Therapies*, Keats Publishing, Inc., New Canaan, 1993.

———. *The Scientific Validation of Herbal Medicine*, Cormorant Books, n.p., 1986.

Murray, Michael T., *The Healing Power of Herbs: The Enlightened Person's Guide to the Wonders of Medicinal Plants*, Prima Publishing, Rocklin, 1992.

Ody, Penelope, *The Complete Medical Herbal*, Dorling Kindersley, London 1993.

Olsen, Cynthia, *Essiac: A Native Herbal Cancer Remedy*, Kali Press, Pagosa Springs, 1996.

Pedersen, Mark, *Nutritional Herbology, Vol. I & II*, Pedersen Publishing, Bountiful, 1987.

Schechter, Steven R., N.D., *Fighting Radiation with Foods, Herbs, & Vitamins*, East West Health Books, Brookline, 1988.

Thomas, Richard, *The Essiac Report: Canada's Remarkable Unknown Cancer Remedy*, The Alternative Treatment Information Network, Los Angeles, 1993.

Tierra, Michael, C.A., N.D., *Planetary Herbology*, Lotus Press, Santa Fe, 1988.

Tyler, Varro E., Ph.D., Sc.D., *Herbs of Choice: The Therapeutic Use of Phytomedicinals*, Pharmaceutical Products Press, New York, 1994.

Weiner, Michael, Ph.D., *Weiner's Herbal*, A Quantum Book, Mill Valley, 1990.

Weiss, Rudolf Fritz, M.D., *Herbal Medicine*, tr. by A. R. Meuss, AB Arcanum, Gothenburg, 1988.

Books on Cancer

Bell, Robert, M.D., *The Prevention and Treatment of Cancer*, Medical Association for the Reduction and Prevention of Cancer, London, n.d.

Binzel, Philip E., Jr., M.D., *Alive and Well: One Doctor's Experience with Nutrition in the Treatment of Cancer Patients*, American Media, Westlake Village, 1996.

Biser, Sam, *The Layman's Course on Killing Cancer*, The Swannanoa Institute, Ltd., 1989.

Boik, John, *Cancer and Natural Medicine, A Textbook of Basic Science and Clinical Research*, Oregon Medical Press, Princeton, Minnesota, 1996.

Clark, Hulda Regehr, *The Cure for All Cancers*, ProMotion Publishing, San Diego, 1993.

Diamond, John W. with Cowden, Lee W. and Goldberg, Burton, *An Alternative Medicine Definitive Guide to Cancer*, Future Medicine Publishing, Inc., Tiburon, 1997.

Gruner, O. Cameron, M.D., *An Interpretation of Cancer*, Health Research, 1947.

Hartwell, Jonathan L., *Plants Used Against Cancer*, Quarterman Publications, Inc., Lawrence, 1982.

Heinerman, John, *The Treatment of Cancer with Herbs*, Biworld Publishers, Orem, 1980.

Hovnanian, Ralph R., *Medical Dark Ages Circa 1984 or Cancer Alternative Therapies' Cure Rates*, Self Published, Evanston, 1985.

Hoxsey, Harry M., N.D., *You Don't Have to Die*, Milestone Books, Inc., New York, 1956.

Morris, Nat, *The Cancer Blackout*, Regent House, Los Angeles, 1977.

Moss, Ralph W., *Cancer Therapy: The Independent Consumer's Guide to Non-Toxic Treatment and Prevention*, Equinox Press, New York, 1992.

_____. *Questioning Chemotherapy*, Equinox Press, New York, 1996.

_____. *The Cancer Industry: The Classic Exposé on the Cancer Establishment*, Equinox Press, 1996.

Jacka, Judy, N.D., *Cancer, A Physical and Psychic Profile*, 1977.

Jones, Eli G., M.D., *Cancer: Its Causes, Symptoms and Treatment*, Therapeutic Publishing Company, Inc., Boston, 1911.

Mohs, Frederic E., B.Sc., M.D., *Chemosurgery: Microscopically Controlled Surgery for Skin Cancer*, Charles C. Thomas Publisher, Springfield, Illinois, 1978.

Nichols, Perry, M.D., *The Value of Escharotics: Medicines which will Destroy Any Living or Fungus Tissue in the Treatment of Cancer, Lupus, Sarcoma or any other Form of Malignancy*, The Roycrofters, East Aurora, 1929.

_____. *The Value of Escharotics: Medicines which will Destroy Any Living or Fungus Tissue in the Treatment of Cancer, Lupus, Sarcoma or any other Form of Malignancy*, The Roycrofters, East Aurora, 1933.

Nuland, Sherwin B., *How We Die: Reflections on Life's Final Chapter*, Alfred A. Knopf, 1994.

Pattison, John, M.D., *Cancer: Its Nature; and Successful and Comparatively Painless Treatment, without the Usual Operation with the Knife*, H. Turner & Co., London, 1866.

Richards, Victor, M.D., *Cancer, The Wayward Cell: Its Origins, Nature, and Treatments*, University of California Press, Berkeley, 1972.

Walters, Richard, *Options: The Alternative Cancer Therapy Book*, Avery Publishing Group, Inc., Garden City Park, 1993.

MEDICAL HISTORY
AND CRITICISM

Coulter, Harris L., *Divided Legacy: A History of the Schism in Medical Thought, Volume I*, Wehawken Book Co., Washington, D.C. 1975.

_____. *Divided Legacy: A History of the Schism in Medical Thought, Volume IV*, North Atlantic Books, 1994.

Ehrenreich, Barbara and English, Deirdre, *Witches, Midwives, and Nurses: A History of Women Healers*, The Feminist Press, New York, n.d.

Fishbein, Morris, M.D., *Fads and Quackery in Healing*, Blue Ribbon Books, New York, 1932.

Grossinger, Richard, *Planet Medicine: From Stone Age Shamanism to Post-Industrial Healing*, North Atlantic Books, 1987.

Ledermann, E. K., Dr., *Medicine for the Whole Person: A Critique of Scientific Medicine*, Element Books, Rockport, 1997.

Robbins, John, *Reclaiming our Health: Exploding the Medical Myth and Embracing the Source of True Healing*, H J Kramer, Tiburon, 1996.

Sjöö, Monica and Mor, Barbara, *The Great Cosmic Mother: Rediscovering the Religion of the Earth*, Harper Collins, 1987, 1991.

Starr, Paul, *The Social Transformation of American Medicine*, Basic Books, Inc., New York, 1982.

Frawley, David, and Lad, Dr. Vasant, *The Yoga of Herbs*, Lotus Press, Santa Fe, 1986.

Frawley, Dr. David, O.M.D., *Ayurvedic Healing*, Passage Press, Salt Lake City, 1989.

Heyn, Birgit, *Ayurvedic Medicine: The Gentle Art of Indian Natural Healing*, translated by David Louch, Thorsons Publishing Group, Ltd., Wellingborough, 1987.

METAPHYSICAL MEDICAL BOOKS

Bott, Victor, M.D., *Anthrosophical Medicine: Spiritual Science and the Art of Healing*, Thorson Publishers, Inc., New York, 1984.

King, Francis X., *Rudolf Steiner and Holistic Medicine*, Nicolas-Hays, Inc., York Beach, 1986.

Strehlow, Dr. Wighard, and Hertzka, Gottfried, M.D., *Hildegard of Bingen's Medicine*, Bear & Co., Santa Fe, 1988.

EASTERN MEDICINE

Burang, Theodor, *The Tibetan Art of Healing*, Watkins Publishing, London, 1974.

Clifford, Terry, *Tibetan Buddhist Medicine and Psychiatry: The Diamond Healing*, Samuel Weiser, Inc., York Beach, 1984.

Donden, Yeshi, Dr., *Health through Balance: An Introduction to Tibetan Medicine*, Snow Lion Publications, Ithaca, 1986.

ARTICLES

Bond, E. Edgar, B.L., M.D., "What's in the Hoxsey Treatment?" *National Health Federation Bulletin*, January, 1961.

Rapgay, Lobsang, Dr., "A Humanistic Approach to Treatment and Management of Cancer," *Tibetan Review*, October, 1983.

Walters, Richard, "Cancer: Do We Already Have a 'Cure'?" *Body, Mind & Spirit*, Jan.-Feb. 1991.

JOURNALS

Bulletin of the Lloyd Library of Botany, Pharmacy and Materia Medica, Reproduction Series, No. 2, *The Indian Doctor's Dispensary Being Father Smith's Advice Respecting Diseases and Their Cure* by Peter Smith, 1812, originally published in Bulletin No. 2, 1901.

Bulletin of the Lloyd Library of Botany, Pharmacy and Materia Medica, Reproduction Series, No. 10, "Hydrastis Canadensis", reprint of the articles entitled "Drugs and Medicines of the North America" (1884), originally published in Bulletin No.10, 1908.

Bulletin of the Lloyd Library of Botany, Pharmacy and Materia Medica, Reproduction Series, No. 11, *Life and Medical Discoveries of Samuel Thomson and a history of the Thomsonian Materia Medica as shown in "The New Guide to Health,"* 1835, originally published in Bulletin No.11, 1909.

Bulletin of the Lloyd Library of Botany, Pharmacy and Materia Medica, Reproduction Series, No. 18, *History of the Vegetable Drugs of the Pharmacopeia of the United States* by John Uri Lloyd, Phar. M., originally published in Bulletin No.18, 1911.

CD-ROM

Christopher, Dr. John R., *The Complete Writings of Dr. John Christopher on CD-ROM*, Herbal Solutions Electronic Publications, Salt Lake City, n.d.

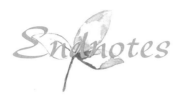

Endnotes

CHAPTER I

1. Victor Richards, M.D., *Cancer: The Wayward Cell*, p. 85.

2. *Hildegard of Bingen's Medicine*, p. xviii.

3. Quoted by John Robbins in *Reclaiming Our Health*, p. 61. Originally from Jessica Mitford, *The American Way of Birth*, Plume, New York, 1993, p. 20.

4. Virgil J. Vogel, *American Indian Medicine*, p. 131.

5. Nat Morris, *The Cancer Blackout*, p. 19.

6. Ibid., p. 27, quoted from Richard Guy's, *Practical Observations on Cancers and Disorders of the Breast, Explaining their Different Appearances and Events, to which are added, One Hundred Cases, Successfully Treated without Cutting*, London, 1762.

7. Ibid., p. 24.

8. Quoted by Wade Boyle in *Pioneers in Nineteenth-Century American Botanical Medicine* and attributed to Otto Juettner, *Daniel Drake and His Followers*, Cincinnati, 1909.

9. Paul Starr, *The Social Transformation of American Medicine*, p. 47.

10. Morris, op. cit., p. 36.

11. Richard Walters in *Body, Mind, & Spirit,* (Jan.-Feb. 1991):11

12. Hartwell, *Plants Used Against Cancer*, lists a publication by Pattison under bloodroot. Pattison is very clear in his book published in 1866 that he used *Hydrastis canadensis*, goldenseal. Hartwell does make several references to Cherokee Indian use of goldenseal. This is confirmed by numerous other sources, such as Vogel and Elkins.

13. Pattison, *Cancer: Its Nature and Successful and Comparatively Painless Treatment without the Usual Operation with the Knife*, H. Turner & Co., London, 1866, p. 88-89.

14. Ibid., p. 103.

15. Ibid., p. 91.

16. Ibid., p. 92.

17. Ibid., p. 93.

18. Druitt, *Surgeon's Vade Mecum*, 6th Edition.

19. *Cancer: Tumors and Malignant Growths both External and Internal Permanently Cured without a Surgical Operation*, New Brunswick, 1905, and *Cancer: Its Causes, Symptoms and Treatment*, published in 1911 by Therapeutic Publishing Company, Inc., Boston.

20. Eli G. Jones, M.D., *Cancer: Tumors and Malignant Growths both External and Internal Permanently Cured without a Surgical Operation*, p. 11.

21. See appendix B for this formula.

22. See appendix B.

23. *The Grape Cure*, p. 115.

24. Nichols, 1933 publication, p. 47.

25. 1950 NCI condition for investigating the Hoxsey treatment.

26. Quoted in the video by Kenny Ausubel, *Hoxsey: When Healing Becomes a Crime*, 1987.

27. Harry Hoxsey, *You Don't Have to Die*, p. 59.

28. Article in *CA—A Cancer Journal for Clinicians*.

29. There is also a more recent version by Loren Biser, Sam Biser's brother.

30. The ingredients for both of these salves are given in appendix B, p. 196-197, along with instructions for preparation of the ointment.

31. *The Layman's Course on Killing Cancer*, 1989, Unit Eight, p. 2.

32. Jane Heimlich, *What Your Doctor Won't Tell You*, p. 45.

33. *Chemosurgery*, p. 5.

34. Walter H. Lewis and Memory P. F. Elvin-Lewis, *Medical Botany*, p. 123.

35. *Cancer Therapy*, p. 163.

CHAPTER 2

36. Op. cit. This case is described on p. 125.
37. See video.
38. Frederic E. Mohs, *Chemosurgery*.

CHAPTER 3

39. *Layman's Course on Killing Cancer,* Unit 8, Lesson 23, p. 9.

40. Penelope Ody, *The Complete Medical Herbal*, p. 42.

41. After writing this, an old herb book published in the last century was loaned to me. It defined escharotics as caustics, either alkalies or acids, that "destroy the vitality of a part by forming a chemical union with one or more of the constituents of the animal body. Their action is afterwards followed by a stimulant reaction." *Materia Medica and Therapeutics including the Preparations of the Pharmacopoeias* of London, Edinburgh, Dublin and [of the United States] by J. Forbes Royle, M.D., F.R.S., 1847, p. 650.

42. Pattison, p. 120.

43. W. John Diamond, M.D., *An Alternative Medicine Definitive Guide to Cancer,* p. 996.

CHAPTER 4

44. Mohs, op. cit., p. 207.

45. See quotation by Druitt on p.15.

CHAPTER 5

46. T. T. Blake, *Cancers Cured without the Use of the Knife*, 1858. Quoted in Morris, p. 28. Blake apparently used an escharotic but, like many before and after, did not divulge his secret formula, saying only that it was purely botanical and contained no poisons.

CHAPTER 6

47. The 1978 edition is available from Charles C. Thomas Publisher in 1978 and is entitled *Chemosurgery*.

48. The video is available from Realidad Productions, P.O. Box 1644, Santa Fe, NM 87504. Tel. 505-982-7019.

49. Harry Hoxsey, *You Don't Have to Die*, p. 159.

50. Though this sometimes happens, it should not generally be expected.

51. In a conversation with her husband, he mentioned that this procedure would have included implant of a radioactive isotope where the one tumor was removed; the second tumor was deemed inoperable

CHAPTER 7

52. Pattison, op. cit, p. 88-89.
53. Ibid., p. 89-90.
54. Ibid, p. 90.

CHAPTER 8

55. Jones, opus cit., p.10.
56. Ibid.
57. Ibid., p.20
58. Ibid., p.20
59. Ibid., p.21
60. Ibid., p.25

61. Ibid., p.28

62. Ibid., p.170

63. Ibid., p.49

64. Ibid., p.259

65. Ibid., p.63

66. Ibid.

67. Ibid., p.260

68. Ibid.

69. Ibid., p.267

70. Ibid., p.87

71. Ibid., p.140

72. Ibid., p.252

73. Ibid., p.142

74. Ibid., p.143

75. Ibid., p.197

CHAPTER 10

76. Yunnan Paiyao is readily available wherever Chinese patent medicines are sold. It comes in several forms, is very inexpensive, and can be safely used to arrest bleeding. There is one tiny pill in each bottle of the powdered form. The pill is for internal use in case of shock or hemorrhaging. The powder can be applied directly to an area that is bleeding or mixed in hot water to stop bleeding. It works remarkably fast and probably belongs in every medicine cabinet.

77. Scargo contains olive oil, peanut oil, lanolin, beeswax, and camphor. It is available from Home Health Products, Inc.in Virginia Beach as well as most health foods stores.

78. Seventh Ray Press carries books by other publishers related to the cancer diet. It also has the author's audio cassette set entitled *Kitchen Doctor*, a must for anyone seriously interested in what to eat and why. Visit the author's Web site: http://www.cancersalves.com for current information.

CHAPTER 11

79. The premixed powders for the bolus are available from The Herb Finder, P.O. Box 2557, St. George, Utah 84771-2557. The telephone number is (435) 652-9593 or 1-800-780-6934; the fax line is (435) 652-3871. They are also available via the author's Web site.

80. See page 199 for the formulae. These can also be ordered from The Herb Finder.

81. Both by patients and foreign gynecologist who saw much potential in the use of these simple remedies.

82. The late Hanna Kroeger recommended that black-strap molasses be used to fill "00" capsules. These were to be inserted vaginally at bedtime for ten days prior to the onset of menstruation. Patients were to douche with apple cider vinegar or chamomile tea in the morning. If not successful the first time, the procedure was to be repeated for ten days before the next cycle.

APPENDIX A

83. Paraphrased from *Song of the Seven Herbs* by Walking Night Bear, 1983.

84. Dorothy Hall, Dorothy Hall's Herbal Medicine, p. 306.

85. Drs. Wighard Strehlow and Gottfried Hertzka, *Hildegard of Bingen's Medicine*, p. 127.

86. Daniel Mowrey, *Herbal Tonic Therapies*, p. 5.

87. Daniel Mowrey, *The Scientific Validation of Herbal Medicine*, p. 57.

88. Charles F. Millspaugh, *American Medicinal Plants*, p. 557.

89. Ralph W. Moss, *Cancer Therapy*, p. 162.

90. Alma R. Hutchens, *Indian Herbology of North America*, p. 82.

91. Ibid, p. 139. Quoted Dr. Charles R. Smart, associate professor of surgery at the University of Utah, who also noted that some patients with advanced disease did not respond to chaparral tea.

92. The Chinese used it much earlier.

93. Moss, op. cit., p. 174.

94. Originally published in *Causæ et Curæ*, 204, 25. Quoted in *Hildegard of Bingen's Medicine*, p. 123, 127, and 129. "Hildegard Medicine" is widely practiced in Germany. Most products described by Hildegard can be obtained from Jura Naturheilmittel, Nestgasse 2, 78464 Konstanz, Germany. Telephone: 07531-31487. Fax: 07531-33403. The violet salve is called *Veilchen-Creme* and the duckweed elixir is called *Wasserlinsen-Elixir*.

95. Ibid, p. 128.

96. In earlier editions, I assumed "pocoon" to be bloodroot, "red puccoon." However, one of my sources stated that all the remedies reported in *Indian Doctor* are Cherokee in origin. In such case, it is possible that the reference is to "yellow puccoon" or goldenseal. See next endnote and note that Daniel Smith was born in an area where bloodroot was used for cancer treatment.

97. From *Indian Doctor*, compiled by Nancy Locke Doane, p. 22. Also found in Daniel Smith's *The Reformed Botanic and Indian Physician*, 1855. Smith was born in the region of Niagara Falls in 1790.

98. I have been unable to identify this plant. One source speculated that it is possibly burdock.

99. Pipsissewa is an Algonquian word. This tea was used by Samuel Thomson.

100. Reported by Walter H. Lewis and Memory P. F. Lewis in *Medical Botany: Plants Affecting Man's Health*, p.

125. The recipe was originally published in *Every Man His Own Doctor*, Williamsburg, 1734. It was reprinted in Annapolis, 1934. Author anonymous.

101. Nat Morris, *The Cancer Blackout*, p. 31.

102. See chapter 7 for procedures using the Pattison preparations.

103. Pattison, op. cit., p. 90-91.

104. Marigold is anti-inflammatory and may help reduce scarring.

105. *The Old Root and Herb Doctor Or the Indian Method of Healing*, 1870.

106. Not identified. This may be an herb or perhaps arsenic?

107. This is a grease that has been used for protecting weapons from rust. My sources indicate that it is still available. One patient suggested using Unpetroleum Jelly.™ Another advised against this substitution. Since this is a healing salve, calendula ointment could be another alternative.

108. Jones, op. cit., p. 91.

109. Ibid, p. 91-92.

110. Mohs, op. cit., p. 5.

111. Hoxsey, op. cit., p. 47.

112. "What's in the Hoxsey Treatment?" by E. Edgar Bond, B.L., M.D., editor of the Journal of *Medical Physical Research*, reprinted from January, 1961, *National Health Federation Bulletin*, San Francisco.

113. Hartwell, *Plants Used Against Cancer*.

114. Available on CD-ROM from The Herb Finder, see endnote no. 79.

115. Dr. John Christopher, *School of Natural Healing*, p. 57.

116. This salve is available from The Herb Finder under the name of *Red Sun Balm*. See endnote no. 79.

117. This ointment is available from The Herb Finder as *German Kermesberro*. See endnote no. 79.

118. Christopher, Op. cit., p. 62.

119. In some sources, Dr. Christopher simply suggested stirring the powdered herbs into the melted cocoa butter and rolling the thickened mixture into boluses.

120. This formula is also available from The Herb Finder. As a bulk tea preparation, it goes by the name of *Partridge Berry Formula* and as capsules, *Change-O-Life Formula*. See endnote no. 79.

121. Sold as *Starwort Formula* by The Herb Finder. See endnote no. 79.

122. Available from The Herb Finder in capsules as PLVC-Ginseng Formula. See endnote no. 79.

123. Christopher, op. cit., p. 58.

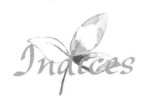

HOMEOPATHIC REMEDIES

The majority of the homeopathic remedies named in this book were cited in connection with the work of Drs. John Pattison and Eli G. Jones. Chapter 7 is devoted to Dr. Pattison and chapter 8 to Dr. Jones. A summary of Dr. Pattison's use of homeopathic remedies appears on page 99 and the remedies used by Jones are described on pages 116-120. For proper use of homeopathic remedies, it is recommended that specialists be consulted.

Poke root, 14, 22, 26, 32, 36-37, 39-43, 47, 89, 95, 98, 107-108, 110, 113, 125, 128-129, 137-138, 173, 176-178, 184, 188, 194-197, 202, 208-209

Poppy, 59

Potatoes, 179

Prickly ash, 95, 193-196, 208

Pseudoginseng, 60, 208

Puccoon, 39, 122, 172-174, 176, 190, 226

Purple cornflower, 111

Purple lady slipper, 100

Queen's delight, 114

Quercus alba, 208

Quinine(s), 100, 110

Raspberry, 199, 208

Red clover, 6, 9, 16, 19, 26, 28, 39, 42, 108, 128-129, 146, 154, 173, 175-176, 185, 189, 191, 194-197, 200-204, 208-209

Red puccoon, 39, 122, 172, 226

Red sandalwood, 15, 39, 208-209

Red sap, 11

Red saunders, 15, 192, 208-209

Red Sun Balm, 22, 39, 87, 147, 176, 196, 227

Rhubarb, 201, 208

Rose, 115, 172, 174, 200, 208

Rose petals, 4

Rue, 187, 208

Rumex crispus, 193, 208

Saffron, 10

Sage, 187, 208

Salicylic acid, 111

Sambucus canadensis, 194

Sanguinaria canadensis, 1, 11, 39, 108, 122, 172, 191-193, 207

Sanguinaria nitrate, 114

Sanguinarin, 113-114

Sanguinarine, 12, 173

Sarcenia purpurea, 100

Sarsaparilla, 180, 196, 199, 202, 208-209

Sassafras, 128, 189, 193, 202

Scrophularia marylandica, 114

Scrophularia nodosa, 17, 26, 127, 193, 207

Scutellaria lateriflora, 101

Scutellarin, 101, 114

Senecio gracilis, 101

Senecionin, 101

Sesame, 152

Sheep's sorrel, 108, 129, 173, 201-203, 208

Siberian ginseng, 199-200, 208

Sinapis arvensis, 207

Slippery elm, 32, 36, 113-114, 137, 150, 192, 198, 201-202, 206, 208-209

Smilax officinalis, 208

Sorrel, 39, 108, 129, 173, 189, 201-203, 208

Speedwell, 39

Spinach, 176

Spigelia, 114

Spike, oil of, 204

Spikenard, 190, 208

Squaw vine, 150, 198-199, 208-209

Staff vine, 110, 208

Starwort, 209, 227

Stillingia sylvatica, 101, 114, 194-196, 208

Stillingin, 101

Stramonium datura, 114, 208

Strawberries, 97

Sweet cicely, 190, 208

Symphytum officinale, 207.

Taraxacum officinale, 207

Tartar, 173

Tartaricum, 173

Termentina, 138

Thistle, 171-172, 179, 201, 207

Thorn apple, 114, 209

Thuja occidentalis, 36, 103, 109-110, 115, 118, 120, 208

Thuja-conium-hydrastis-phytolacca, 115

Thujone, 171

Thyme, 60

Tormentil, 187, 208

Trifolium compound, 16, 127, 154, 175-176, 195-196

Trifolium pratense, 175, 185, 208

Turkey corn, 60, 110, 208

Turmeric, 32, 62, 65, 125, 129-130, 132, 135-136, 139, 143-144, 146, 173, 180-181, 184, 203-205, 208

Turnip, 150

Unguent resinosum flavae, 95, 98

Uva ursi, 199-200, 208-209

Vervain, 190, 208

Viburnin, 101

Viburnum opulus, 101, 115, 207

Viola spp, 3, 208

Violets, 3, 28, 39, 41, 169-170, 187

Wahoo, 208-209

Walnut, 87, 129, 160, 198, 204, 208

Walnuts, 200

Wasserlinsen-elixir, 226

Watercress, 201

White American hellebore, 94

White oak, 209

White pond lily, 112

White *pinus canadensis*, 115

White pond lily, 112

Willow, 60, 129-130, 205

Wintergreen, 32, 60, 111, 196, 204, 208

Witch hazel, 47, 114, 131-133, 192

Wormwood, 208

Woundwort, 171

Yarrow, 3, 16-17, 26, 125, 127, 130, 169-172, 187, 208

Yellow dock, 150, 173, 180, 190, 198, 200, 208-209

Yellow puccoon, 39, 122, 174, 226

Xanthoxylum fraxineum, 95, 99, 101

Zingiber officialis, 207

General Index

OTHER PUBLICATIONS BY THE AUTHOR

Stress: the Cause of Disease
The Elements: Constitutional Type and Temperament
Cancer: The Psychospiritual Pathology of Disease
Immunity
Lunar Consciousness

FORTHCOMING

Fate: Destiny or Karma?
Shadows on the Soul

AUDIO CASSETTE SERIES

Kitchen Doctor
Adrenal Exhaustion
Cancer Salves
The Elements
Astroendocrinology

AVAILABLE FROM:

Seventh Ray Press

P.O. Box 235
SUQUAMISH, WASHINGTON 98392

FAX: 1-888-FAX-HEAL OR 1-360-779-9677

WEBSITES

http://www.cancersalves.com
http://www.kitchendoctor.com